Discussing child and adolescent mental health nursing

Discussing child and adolescent mental health nursing

by

Sandy Fitzgibbon and Dean–David Holyoake

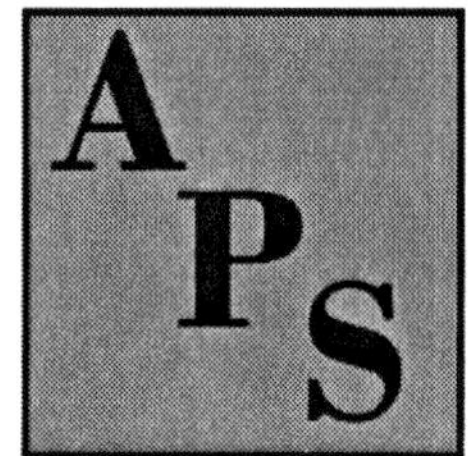

APS Publishing, The Old School, Tollard Royal, Salisbury, Wiltshire, SP5 5PW; www.apspublishing.co.uk

British Library Cataloguing in Publication Data
A catalogue record for this book is available from the British Library

ISBN 1 9038771 5 6

Printed in the UK by Selwood Printing Ltd. West Sussex

Contents

Acknowledgements

It is important that the authors acknowledge the great contribution Martin Pursey (also known as our friendly critic or MP) made during the writing of this book. As a colleague with experience in adolescent mental health nursing his careful reading of drafts and his useful comments helped shape the re-thinking of the topics.

Rethinking child and adolescent mental health nursing: A postmodern perspective

❖ It is said that the (M)odernist individual is self-controlled, unitary, discrete, orderly, orientated towards thought, language and representation.

➢*The postmodern is 'uncontrolled*, decentred *multiplicitous, transgressive*, orientated towards ***affect***, ***image*** and ***simulation***

(Michael, 1990: 77)

(The capital (M) as in (M)odernism indicates the theory, or critical approach; modern (with a lower case m) indicates modern in the ordinary sense, i.e. contemporary of our time, current, or even trendy).

Opening dialogue

Introduction

When we started writing this book we made two assumptions. First, (because we both have a background in child and adolescent mental health nursing), we believed we shared similar views. Second, that any conflicting views could be easily overcome and utilised in our writing. However, we soon discovered that we had many differences which belonged to our shared culture. While not wanting to explain all the differences encountered, we should mention the major difference of our gender emerged early on and guided our introduction to the use of dialogues. In an attempt to identify patterns of difference and make connections, the dialogues presented in each chapter are given in the hope that they will help set the context. The dialectical method of inquiry was utilised by Plato as a way to record the wisdom of spoken thought. As a method, it maintains the Socratic belief that philosophy should be alive and always critical. The dialogues presented throughout this book are taken from actual transcripts of the authors as they drafted this book.

Sandy: Child and adolescent mental health nursing has evolved over a number of years and in a number of ways, which has led to some confusion about what place we have as nurses in the multi-professional teams. This evolution is a construction. It isn't a natural phenomenon. It's a construction of ideas, attitudes and beliefs about what the nursing role should be. It includes how children, their families and other professionals view our role.

Dean: This idea of evolution reflects the way in which some nursing academics are now beginning to question our traditional role and the assumptions we have regarding nursing, a role that has always had its foundation in the biomedical model of science. This is traditionally viewed as belonging to a Modernist period of scientific progress. The postmodern age is more about questioning practice rather than prescribing it.

Sandy: I was expecting you to want to write a book based very much in the positivist and reductionist genre, a book that supported the advancement of scientific progress based upon research findings.

Dean: Scientific progress reflects societal changes, so I am wondering if, in this book, we should be questioning practice rather than prescribing it.

Sandy: Oh! That's a relief. I thought that you might expect us to present a perspective based in reductionism and, as that has already been contributed to very well by other authors, I think we need to offer some alternative views to those of the majority if we are to advance child and adolescent nursing practice.

Dean: Yes, but we should remember that child mental health nurses have a history that is bound up in the medical model and I question if you are suggesting that we should abandon this?

Sandy: No certainly not, we need to respect and recall our historical roots, but also let's not fool ourselves into believing that our role is to follow the medical viewpoint to the end. Medics already understand this model better than we can and, if we are to work together effectively as part of a multi-professional group, we need to bring to the team a different view of the mental health of children and teenagers.

Dean: OK. I can see that if this were the case perhaps our clients might receive a more holistic approach to care. Even so I think that we still need to understand the medical model in some way in order to be able to work closely with doctors.

Sandy: I don't disagree with that, but I also believe that we don't have to abandon one model in favour of another. We don't have to take the reductionist perspective of either/or; we can hold the view of both/and.

Dean: Sounds interesting, but in compiling this book where do you suggest our focus should be?

Sandy: What I am suggesting is that it should be a modern nursing book regulated by philosophies that reflect the beliefs of (M)odernism and postmodernism; you know, reflecting the contemporary age we live in. However, thinking about (M)odernism and post-modernism isn't as easy as contemplating the symptoms of a depressed child or young person.

Dean: I follow you OK, but does it need to be so hyper?

Sandy: It's hyper, as you call it, due to us living and nursing in a hyper reality. The way we think, communicate, and understand our reality can be said to be about living in a reality of the mass-produced representations which legitimise our roles. We are products of our reality, but that isn't as natural as we may think.

Dean: So what is it that makes child and adolescent mental health nursing (M)odern and postmodern?

Sandy: That's a huge question and one I am sure cannot be answered simply, but perhaps we should explore it throughout this book. As you mention it now, I think what we need to do is to try to separate out the modern and the postmodern before attempting integration.

Dean: Aren't they the same with just one following the other?

Sandy: If you mean a progression is involved, then possibly. There is a lot of confusion about where the two separate or even if they do. To use your language, postmodernism could be just hyper-modernism, on the other hand it could be a distinct age. We know that postmodernist criticism has challenged the way we view knowledge and scientific-based fact. We take it for granted that (M)odernism is about industrialisation, mass production, consumerism, capitalism, and free market economics, and these can all be seen reflected in the nursing and therapeutic models.

Dean: So is postmodernism just more of the same, but at a later date? From what you have said it seems to me that (M)odernism is a sort of being; it is how we are today, how we nurse, and it's all around us. Postmodernism is a way of doing, a method for teasing out (M)odernism and the way it chafes at what we do and the way we do it.

Sandy: Yes and no. It can't be an age that flows out of (M)odernism because this would be an example of the grand narrative mythology criticised by postmodernism. To confuse you further, it is often seen as belonging to the same age, but it demonstrates disillusionment with universals. It tries to highlight how oppositions in thought and language have been neglected and it is this neglect which provides evidence for structures and discourses in the way society has perceived reality.

Dean: All right, let me have a go at explaining how I have perceived it so far. What we're saying is that it's about the way we represent ourselves as modern; the way we are a clean, efficient machine. So it's not necessarily a rejection or denial of what nursing has done so far. We have reached this point in time and are now, and only now, able to re-think about the ways we represent, reproduce, and legitimise ourselves. Namely, advancing nursing practice.

Sandy: Yes. This is the professional project.

Dean: You mean the way nursing perceives itself in reality.

Sandy: Absolutely; but twentieth century thought has emphasised the importance of language. Only in this (M)odernist era has language been able to provide the postmodernism critique. So post-modernism is also a development or a result of (M)odernism in more than mere name.

Dean: And that is the focus for our book. This needs to be reflected in the content of the book.

Sandy: Well, we need to set the (M)odern scene and include postmodernism thinking, then move forward towards the (M)odernist project.

Dean: And critique (M)odernist concepts before attempting to draw some themes together.

Sandy: Well, setting the Modern scene is about doing the usual thing. We need to do this to argue that nursing belongs to the modern, and that it has a knowledge base which reflects the wider thought of western culture, philosophy, and metaphysics.

Dean: It should also include ideas about the main themes of this modern era... you know, like child-centred caring and expanding practice.

Sandy: And postmodernism?

Dean: The second section is about how the (M)odernist can be related to a postmodern critique. A sort of example of the actual techniques academics have used to understand Modernism.

Sandy: In that case, the 'Modernist project' is about the way nursing is modernist and relates to a modernist reality.

Dean: What we're actually going to do is re-think child and adolescent nursing aren't we? I mean we're all so used to accepting that the position we find ourselves in today is natural, it's easy to ignore how nursing generally has gone through loads of change. It's about modernism isn't it. You know, looking back and reflecting upon what we have already achieved.

Sandy: Yes, we need to examine the current nursing of children. This is to do with modernism because to reflect on past practice is to advance nursing practice.

Dean: Advanced nursing practice being about pushing boundaries and developing new ways in which nurses in child and adolescent mental health will pioneer new roles and approaches. It's a sort of individual thing then? (M)odernism is about a general approach to self-critical reflection as individuals and a profession. What do we think are some important themes that need to run throughout the book?

Sandy: I believe we need to start with reviewing the knowledge base of nursing and locate it within a modernist view, and then consider the great science and art debate.

Dean: We need to include in this major theme the concepts of child-centred caring. For example, what is this concept? It sounds rather motherly to me, but what we should be representing within our therapeutic relationships with our clients?

Sandy: Moving onto the 'Modernist project', we need to consider professional boundaries and power.

Dean: We're really talking about the way nursing identifies itself and the boundaries of practice that have been built upon cultural perspectives and assumptions.

Sandy: Yes, and what can follow from this are expert views and advanced nursing practice.

Dean: We should concluded this major theme with consideration of Attachment. You are often pushing the need to understand the theories of Attachment but perhaps we could consider this through the nature of power structures.

Sandy: Another important point that is part of the third theme is about authority. It's about Bion and Winnicot's holding and is actioned by putting down the guidelines and boundaries for children to feel safe and secure, so they can trust us.

Dean: The way we use language and the concepts of nursing can be said to direct the way we view the way we practise.

Sandy: Yes, it's about exploring the routines and ideas which direct the building of knowledge.

Dean: It's never that black and white though, is it? After all, we're not coming from a deterministic position. It's a sort of existential or free will philosophical position in which the child and young person is in the centre. This is about the **interpretivist paradigm**; it's about the subjective experience of health and illness.

Sandy: Well, it doesn't have to be, you know. It should highlight that a hospital admission is only a phase of treatment; it's not the be all and end all for the child or the young person. This brings to mind the next topic, the therapeutic milieu. We need to consider the separation of a young person or child from his or her parents and the effects of institutions on the child and the care he/she receives.

Dean: Then we need to draw all our ideas and questions together to help us to move toward the new Post, postmodern perspective

We have not written this book in order to explain the role and function of nurses in child, adolescent and mental health nursing, but in the hope that it will contribute to further questioning of your own knowledge and awareness of the assumptions, which you make due to historical initiatives. Meanwhile, we need to continue to search for knowing how best to care for the mental health of children and teenagers.

Sandy FitzGibbon and Dean-David Holyoake

Re-thinking child and adolescent mental health nursing: A postmodernist perspective

Introduction

The aim of this book is to contribute to the child and adolescent mental health nursing debate with something different, something post-modern and post-Health Advisory Service (HAS, 1995). By post-modern we mean something that is not automatically accepting of the dominant theories of science, historicism and the attempt, in this (M)odernist era, to glean grand universal narratives from reality using a model of the natural sciences. We view postmodernism as both a development and a result of (M)odernist epistemology of which nursing *per se* is unavoidably a part. Thus, postmodernism means questioning the idea of 'progress', the plausibility of global explanations of conduct, and the idea that we, as nurses, practise and care for the mental health of young people in the spirit of the age of purposive rationality, as we have always assumed and been taught. This does not mean that the book is anti-medical, positivist, reductionist, (M)odernist, or empirical; rather, it highlights a conviction by the authors, and many other nurses, that issues of child-centred care, holism, and phenomenological/ existential philosophies could provide alternatives and strengthen the science and ideas of what it is to be human that are already in place. It is true that the desire to 'advance nursing' and give it an expanded role within the dominant psychiatric model (with its biological, mechanistic and disease-focussed approach) sits comfortably within the realms of modernist epistemology, ontology, and methodology. For postmodern thought, however, this comfort is not so easy to explain. These are philosophical issues (holism, knowledge, professionalism, ideology, labelling) that distinguish what is fundamental to nursing. Throughout the book, these concepts will be explored further, because their importance in advancing a re-think of child and adolescent mental health nursing will be central. It is argued, as a central premise of this book, that the strength of postmodernist thought in nursing is its ability to locate and expose the underlying metaphysical and professional assumptions about 'progress', which have hitherto guided nursing theory of mentally young people. By doing so, it is hoped that, ultimately, practice will benefit.

The themes that run throughout the book are not necessarily concerned with new issues, rather they will be analysed from a postmodern perspective. The first issue of 'Setting the Modernist Scene' highlights the courageous attempts nursing scholars have made to create a unified knowledge base of nursing. This knowledge base, shaped by a modernist ethos for order, objectivity, and a compulsion by man to dominate his nature, concerns the philosophical debate of how we know what we know. This is, in itself, an arduous task attempted by few if any contemporary textbooks on child and adolescent mental health nursing. Rather, the more comfortable acceptance of modernist thought and its positivist framework has always ensured that the employment of classifications, diagnosis, and a structure of treatment modalities of nursing care (for example, how to care for a schizophrenic) will never be redundant in practice. This book argues that, although we may find it sometimes nauseous, annoying, and irritating, the uncertainty of fragmented postmodern thought, as offered in this book, can serve as a pointer to relevant alternatives. As noted in the preceding dialogue by the authors, just trying to locate such a perspective has proved difficult. This is partly due to the fact that, because nursing has been dominated for so long by a positivist and (M)odernist ideology, it is almost impossible to conceive of any nursing thought outside the cause and effect relationship. By positivist ideology, the authors refer to that framework of theory and value-laden belief, which is considered by mainstream psychiatry to be fundamental to how we should view children and young people's development and care needs. However, it has seldom been acknowledged in other textbooks on the topic of nursing care. It is important to note that, although the authors are not crudely anti-medical, we do consider psychiatry to be a distinct and separate discourse. Psychiatry is a social construction that has attempted to employ epistemologies and methodologies of the natural sciences to the study of humanity in a (M)odernist project. In particular, we argue that psychiatry is, in fact, concerned with power and its interplay between social actors and their everyday life experiences. It has failed in its task of providing a 'truthful' knowledge base. Instead, it has simply provided a neat and tidy conceptual framework founded upon trembling metaphysical foundations and shaky psychiatric ideology. The term 'metaphysics' is defined as a way of thinking not necessarily based upon a priori or empirical data. It is concerned with modern rational and logical thought usually associated in nursing with models of practice.

There are a number of theses central to postmodern thought, which we offer to promote the re-thinking of child and adolescent mental health nursing. They are used as a foundation or 'starter' in an area of philosophical thought which, unfortunately, is anything but inherently ordered. It is traditional in this type of book to spend a considerable amount of time giving historical accounts of where nursing has come from. This in itself demonstrates the obsession with order, universally accepted knowledge, and a manmade interpretation of the considered 'truth'. However, this is not the case with this book. Instead, the reader is asked to consider the ideas that have dominated the book's development and are presented at the end of this introduction below. It is hoped that this will act as a sort of pause, so that the reader gets a sense of the philosophical issues and themes into which they will be expected to leap. Philosophically significant topics, such as 'Language as a commentator' and 'Mental illness as a manmade construction', are woven through several chapters to provide a post-modern critique (Critiquing Modernist Concepts: A Postmodernist Project). Apart from the broad theses listed below, a thesis for each of the four sections and every chapter is given at the start of each; together they form a map of thought which the reader may or may not find a useful guide. This is an important issue, because we certainly don't expect every reader to agree with the authors. However, we do intend to start a debate, one that in the postmodern tradition of disappointment with universals will be beneficial for the dismantling of discourse and the deconstruction of assumed metaphysical beliefs.

The term 'mentally ill young people' is used to refer to those who have or will come into contact with all four official tiers of health care provision. It is by this very contact that they are labelled mentally ill. The distinction between children and adolescents throughout this book refers to the often quoted developmental milestones—physical, mental and social—which are taken for granted and, indeed, often stressed within the (M)odernist view of things. Although not wishing to call particular attention to this, the authors, where possible, have attempted to use the term 'young people' to include all that is **not** developmentally specific. The distinction between the two groups in this developmental and pragmatic sense is acknowledged.

Theses that guided development of the book

- One does not have to scratch too far below the surface to understand that struggles about ideology, power, and knowledge are inseparable from all human relations, language, and thought. This is a central concern and posit of postmodernist thought
- the postmodern critique is both a nuisance and uncomfortable for readers and writers because it does not provide any conceptual wholes, as provided by the (M)odernist project
- nursing by its very nature helps to determine the culture within which it is practised; it is also very much a product of that culture
- as such, nursing is a (M)odernist project, primarily concerned with progress
- the notions of professionalism and the rise of nursing specialisms are part of the same progress project in which nursing has attempted to create and define a role
- advancement and autonomy are reflections of the ideological and power relations invested in nursing progress. As such, the advanced nurse practitioner (ANP) is seen as the very best the culture of nursing can offer at present
- the knowledge base of nursing is fundamentally a (M)odernist concern related to issues of power
- the language used specifically in the care domain and in human history is not just a vehicle for speech, it is laden with assumptions, power, and oppositional assumptions from which it cannot be separated, even when it claims 'objectivity'
- the Enlightenment philosophies of humanism and holism shared by many competing theoretical rivals within health care merely reflect the way nursing has adopted and is entwined within the (M)odernist project
- humanism and holism as foundations for practice are ideologically, politically, and culturally determined even though nursing has invested in them as being scientific and progressive
- human science even if it is concerned with the 'nature' of humanity in the modern sense cannot be studied with the methods proper to natural science
- the speciality of child and adolescent mental health nursing is dominated by a psychiatric and general medical nursing discourse
- it legitimises its position by appealing to the nature of the materials it uses (young people)

- Post-modernism identifies that (M)odernism legitimises its dominance via self-legitimisation. This secures a firmer entrenchment of modernist critique in its area of competence
- Postmodernist critiques highlight that humanism, holism and positivism (like any other philosophy) rely upon metaphysical foundations which are themselves open to critique. For example, humanism and a full acknowledgement of patients' freewill do not go hand in hand when nursing young people and children
- child and adolescent mental health nursing has boundaries that always take into account the nature of the unique nature of the subjects, e.g. age and development issues. However, child and adolescent mental health nursing derives largely from the models of underlying metaphysics of adult psychiatry, and relies on them to order practice and derive the constraints which place it in a wider reality
- the Health Advisory Report (HAS Report, 1995) provides a platform from which nursing young people can be re-thought and perhaps advanced.

Section I: Setting the modern scene

Aims for this section :

(1) To emphasise that our current view of nursing reality is dominated by positivism and metaphysical assumptions usually applied to the natural sciences;

(2) To introduce the notion that child and adolescent mental health nursing, as with all nursing, has an inevitable relationship to our own century's understanding and knowledge of man; and

(3) To explore the way nursing has attempted to define and reinvent itself with reference to holism, the nature of caring, the ownership of a distinct scientific nursing knowledge base and the philosophy of humanism.

Chapter 1
The knowledge base of nursing

"Now what I want is Facts. Teach these boys and girls nothing but Facts. Facts alone are wanted in life. Plant nothing else, and root out everything else ... Stick to the Facts, Sir!"

Charles Dickens (Hard Times: 1)

Dialogue

Dean: We've got to set the scene in this chapter. We've got to place child and adolescent nursing within its philosophical, theoretical and scientific foundations. You know, its (M)odernist position.

Sandy: We need to mention holism don't we...?

Dean Yeah, but what I was thinking is that this chapter has to describe how nursing can be located within a (M)odernist view and then how post-modernism is a set of reactions to twentieth century (M)odernism, which can be utilised to critique nursing and the philosophies, such as humanism and holism, that we take for granted.

Sandy: You mean introduce the ideas of structuralism and phenomenology as opposed to positivism?

Dean: Yeah, to demonstrate that modernism has resulted in alternative paradigms of thought.

Sandy: Well, I think we need to define what we mean by paradigm and meta-paradigm to start with, and then give a general description of how it is possible to re-think child mental health nursing.

Dean: You mean...?

Sandy: I mean that most other texts on child and adolescent mental health nursing seem to just accept that science is about proving facts. You know, a child has temper tantrums because he has experienced bad parenting, etc.

Dean: You mean the cause and effect argument?

Sandy: Exactly, and we know that issues are far more complex than that and should be viewed more holistically, you know, taking into account the ontology and epistemology of illness from a more feminine and constructivist paradigm, which moves it away from trying to prove the cause, to understanding the phenomenological experience.

Dean: So the premise for this chapter is that the knowledge base of nursing is usually viewed from a positivist and natural science dominated paradigm except that there is now some interest in phenomenological approaches. This has failed to allow alternative ways of critically examining nursing because everything has to be concerned with rationales, evaluating output and researching practice in terms of logic and cause and effect. The use of postmodernist critique highlights these issues of dominant discourse.

Thesis of this chapter

- Nursing is (M)odernist because of its relation to technological, theoretical and sociological advances. It cannot be separated from the culture in which it practices
- The modernist project of providing a complete all embracing knowledge base for nursing has failed
- Postmodernist critique does not attempt to provide answers to creating an all embracing universal knowledge base; instead, it highlights its impossibility and uselessness for nursing
- Science and art cannot be divided as is often thought in mainstream positivist science. If nursing wishes to adopt holism as a guiding philosophical notion, then this is a poignant consideration

Background and aims

This chapter aims to explore some of the philosophical movements in twentieth century critical thought and consider their theoretical relation to child and adolescent nursing. It might seem unusual to present such abstract ideas about something that is considered as down-to-earth as nursing ill young people, but these philosophical debates about human action and society have raged, and will continue to rage regardless of nursing's wish to participate or not. It is suggested throughout this book that the functionalist notions of society and the relationship with the individual, be they nurse or young person, have an evolutionary overtone. As such, theories of social evolution view the development of science as being crucial to the development of human culture. This notion of progress, and the recent development in this century of psychological and sociological paradigms of thought from which nursing draws, can be viewed as a result of modernity. The primary study of 'natural man' since the renaissance has been superseded by the study of 'social man' in relation to what Durkheim (1858–1917) called, ‘a social fact’. This includes the turning of people into subject matter for science, including the social relationships between them. Max Weber’s whole work (1864–1920), according to Smith (1997: 554), was directed towards answering the question: ‘Which social factors have brought about the rationalisation of Western civilisation?’ The disciplines of sociology and psychology were born of a modern age to provide terms and a language for an engaged response to this modern Western civilisation. (M)odernity exhibits an overwhelming commitment to goal-orientated action, the organisation of social affairs by rational means for the rational ends of efficiency, order and material satisfaction (Smith, 1997: 561). This likening of human groups to organisms, dynamics, and hierarchies of parts was performed as far back as Plato. Twentieth century nursing only has to look back as far as the functionalist school of thought of this century.

The search for logical understanding about the social nature of man has, in the modernist sense, been a project of all these paradigms of scientific thought. How we view ourselves and nursing care today is usually seen as being either determined by evolution or as a direct result of scientific progress. It is assumed that in another 100 years, nursing will be even more advanced. However, these are assumptions based upon a belief that we can truly know the nature of reality and that there are predictable patterns of human behaviour waiting to be found. This is the current belief advocated by most nurses and shored up by an ideology of psychiatry. In contrast, the postmodern thought belonging to the second half of this century is a critique of the assumptions endorsed by (M)odernism. Although postmodern thought shares the same cultural and historical developments and is ultimately related to modernity, it has no truck with the predictable fixed and solid theoretical certainties that are supposed to be the modernist Utopia. As noted by Donna Haraway (1988), ‘The further I get in describing…postmodernism…the more nervous I get’. As such, the important contributions of postmodernist thought discussed throughout this book represent philosophical concepts that we maintain do have significance in nursing young people. First, it is argued that nursing has a relationship with (M)odernism and second, that the (M)odernist mode of understanding the world has created nursing; nursing is not an autonomous self creation. In order to progress this argument it will be necessary to explain the notions of paradigm and meta-paradigm insofar as they apply to nursing, and this is discussed in the following pages.

The paradigm of nursing

The paradigm of nursing is an assortment of concepts, terms, and inferences with which nursing academics have attempted to create a unifying theory of nursing, and provide a comprehensive way of defining nursing, incorporating critical social theory as well as the science of nursing. The actuality remains, however, that such a desire is far from being achieved as a universality of nursing. The notion of specialisms within nursing, with their more focussed application, tends to follow the positivist model that a unified view, similar to that of medicine and adopted by psychiatry, could benefit nursing, theoretically. It is with this in mind that this chapter's ultimate aim is to provide a sketch pad introduction to an alternative complex set of reactions to the positivist notion that knowledge can be categorised in certain ways in order to universalise it. Therefore, it is first necessary to consider the dominant theoretical discourses, which include positivism, that drive nursing in child and adolescent mental health nursing, as opposed to the uncertainty of postmodernist alternative views now emerging. The aims of this chapter are:

1. Consider the theoretical position of the paradigm and meta-paradigm of nursing in child and adolescent mental health nursing;
2. Highlight the significance of twentieth century thought for re- thinking child and adolescent mental health nursing; and
3. Discuss the philosophical concepts of holism.

Introduction

The discipline of child and adolescent mental health nursing has gone through something of a metamorphosis in recent years. The development of regional and local tier services heralds the beginning of a post-HAS Report (1995) era that has provided a perplexing and unusual environment as the profession continues to seek its own identity. The whole profession is fatigued with debate about educational needs, philosophical paradigms, holism versus reductionism, tier service provision and the more recent development of advancing/expanding nurse practice. These issues are only part of the equation as nursing at the turn of the twentieth century strives towards an all graduate profession and has the aim of standing next to medicine and, therefore, psychiatry as an equal, so changing the balance of power between the caring trades. In every nursing journal, there is evidence to suggest a clear shift, both in the nature of debates within nursing and in its relationship with other disciplines. At one level, nurses and therapists are becoming more and more receptive to the whole domain of cultural theory, philosophy and sociology—as a result more and more questions regarding the nature of nursing are being asked and engaged. The belief that by advancing nursing practice we can build a Utopia with unquestioned foundations is a troubling assumption, but one that may have relevance to child and adolescent mental health nursing. It is perhaps no coincidence that this book appears at the end of the twentieth century, a period we might mark with a moment of calm. Whereas the twentieth century began with a note of exhilaration, with inspiring calls to a progressive and glorious future, our century is ending on a note of reflection. For our profession, it began and developed with ideals of a new method of caring for mentally ill young people and closes with a 're-thinking' of caring. Therefore, we look backwards in order to move forward. We need to question the philosophical metaphysics, which have raised eyebrows and consider their implications for the future care of the mental health of young people.

It is important to point out the distinction between that which is rooted in old and accepted metaphysical beliefs about nursing practice and that which belongs to the postmodern. In the past, professionals believed that individuality and, therefore, child-centred care was/is the way forward out of the era of grand universal diagnosis and classification systems of disease and perceptions of illness, which belong to the established positivist paradigm of science. It is important to point out the growing widespread questioning of various concepts and the value judgements on which contemporary child health care has been founded, such as the role of the nuclear family, the role of mothering, attachment issues and individuality. These assumptions, which are the foundations of much of our nursing practice, are being questioned in a way which could loosely be termed 'postmodern'. At present, the speciality lacks a knowledge base and epistemology that is truly nursing led. Nurses generally go along with two assumptions: first, that mental illness is a biological reality and, second, all young people identified as mentally ill can be treated within fixed frameworks of diagnosis, treatment and follow up. Moreover, these can all be re-framed in different geographical areas, which risks putting individual personhood well behind the need to prioritise resources. This is a product of modernity.

If we take as our first premise that all children and young people must necessarily be treated as individuals (a belief nursing has upheld for forty years) it is necessary to provide a distinction between the postmodern and the positivist view of science. To do this, readers should be aware of the term 'paradigm' because philosophical issues related to differing paradigms are central to much of the debate within social science, science and philosophy. As noted by Kvale (1990: 20) it was Kuhn's, *The Structure of Scientific Revolutions* (1970) 'that provided the strongest attack on foundationalist thought'. For child and adolescent nursing to open itself up to such impulses need not be thought of as an indulgence. On the contrary, child and adolescent mental health nursing is not the autonomous art and science it sometimes perceives itself to be. Nursing is part of the complete web of social and political concerns, and failing to understand this is a failure to understand the full philosophical and social impact of postmodernist thought in our profession. Furthermore, only an extreme positivist would claim that our concept of nursing is not mediated by consciousness. The refusal to address the ways in which this mediation takes place is a refusal to address the deep questions of child and adolescent mental health nursing. These are questions about the way nurses and young people view themselves, knowledge and the gaining of knowledge. These concern ontology, epistemology and methodology, as noted by Draper (1993) who also provides a concise definition of these three important concepts. An understanding of them is necessary in order to move forward.

Ontology, epistemology and methodology

The ontological debate concerns the fundamental nature of social reality for the individual. There are a number of ways it can be thought of in philosophical terms. Draper states that the realist believes social reality to be an external phenomenon that impinges upon the consciousness of the individual from without. For example, when a young person is faced with school pressure, bullying and family difficulties, these are seen as being external forces that exist in reality for the young person; they are forces that affect the way they feel about themselves, others and their environment. However, there is a second view known as nominalism, which considers the way individuals construct reality by way of cognition. This is the constructivist approach (not to be confused with the constructionist approach, which studies culture and social structures). From the constructionist perspective, how one young person views his/her existence is based upon how he/she perceives his/her reality. So in the mind of the young person who feels herself being bullied, it is no use for even a well-informed observer to say 'objectively, dear, this isn't bullying': it is the victim's understanding of what constitutes bullying that is the issue. Immediately, it becomes more apparent that there is no philosophical general consensus regarding the issue of ontology: i.e. it will be difficult to assert 'bullying exists here' or to demonstrate 'that is not a case of bullying'. In looking at the events of social and mental life, this uncertainty about the existence of the things we study is a constant theme.

The epistemological debate concerns the nature of knowledge. It has two major contributors. Firstly, the positivist, who believes that the search for regularities and casual relationships will eventually lead to objective truth (Draper, 1993). This is evident in most biological, pathological and medical science. Opposed to this view in the epistemological arena is the antipositivist group of theories, which broadly make up the constructivist and postmodern constructionist theories. As noted by Draper (1993), these view the world as essentially relativistic and state that it can only be understood in terms of the subjective meanings held by the individuals whose activities are the focus of study. The two are non-compatible epistemologically speaking, but confusion occurs due to possible ontological and methodological similarities. Positivism strives for scientific certainty utilising mostly quantitative methods of research, such as checklists, random sampling and double blind trials. At its most ambitious, science claims to advance knowledge rigorously, by insisting that hypotheses are tested by falsification, i.e. by making daring predictions that might be disproved by a single negative instance. This is an idealised picture of actual research method. The use of qualitative methods, such as in-depth interviews and techniques derived from anthropology and ethnography, are mostly used within nursing due to their ability to explore the subjective. These methods are antipositivist. They do not emphasise systematic protocols or testing theory via the use of hypothesis.

Traditionally, nursing discourse has largely imitated the discourse of medicine and psychiatry. In general, it has been dominated by debates that revolve around questions of positivism and science. In these debates, science has seized the moral high ground with arguments that seek their authority or legitimacy in terms of the supposed superiority of 'scientific fact'. Such debates have often been confined to 'signs of symptoms'. In a similar vein to the rational way Descartes and his followers tried to reduce all certainty to the individual, medicine and psychiatry reduce certainty to an empirical diagnosis. Nursing discourse can be said to have been licensed by, and allowed to operate on the sufferance of the medical and psychological disciplines. As such, child and adolescent mental health nursing is a product of a way of thinking. It is not a way of fact or certainty. It is a synthesised paradigm of thought which needs to be examined so that we can answer the question, 'What is going on here?'

The paradigm

The concept of a paradigm is essential to an understanding of modern nursing philosophy and theory. A paradigm is an overall framework embracing determinants of behaviour: *perceptual-cognitive* (such as attributes and premises), *axiological* (such as values and beliefs), and *cognitive-transactional* (such as motivations and interactive modes). A paradigm expresses a self-consistent world view, a social construction of reality (Berger, 1977) widely taken for granted by the members of a community, such as mental health nurses caring for young people; most of whom are aware only to a limited extent of the logic and, according to Perlmutter and Trist (1986), metaphysics that underlie their actions is implicit rather than explicit in what they feel and think, and in the courses of action they undertake. For example, it is expected in the assessment of a young person that nurses will make a detailed family history (usually similar to those done by medical personal), and an account of family details, reasons for referral, safety issues, physical, social and spiritual needs. It is a routine assumption that nurses' reasons for doing so are, of course, beneficial to the young person, to the provision of his care and even to his family. Few realise that such routine belongs within the paradigm of nursing, generally, due to its deep philosophical foundations of positivism. Paradigms, although not new, are often misunderstood.

The term 'paradigm' was first used by Thomas Kuhn (1962) to describe a set of scientific and metaphysical beliefs that make up a theoretical framework within which scientific theories can be tested, evaluated and, if necessary, revised. It changed the way traditional positivist science is viewed. For example, the belief that childhood is a distinct transitional period of development challenged a long held view that children were just little and younger adults. Scientifically, this was established by the work of Erikson, Piaget, child psychoanalysis and behavioural theory. It is now considered fact and viewed as a part of the linear progression through which science tests hypotheses in its quest for the ultimate universal truths. However, as noted by Enc (1995: 557) the notion of paradigms strongly challenges this logical empiricist's view of how scientific theory changes; that is, the belief that facts have to be superseded by new facts when they are proved wrong and, therefore, create a revision in our ever increasing knowledge of reality. This positivist view has attempted to provide a universal and unifying perspective to science at a macro and micro level. Kuhn argues that this does not actually happen. Instead, he argues that one scientific paradigm is replaced by another in a paradigm revolution. Each paradigm contains a specific area of scientific interest, such as nursing. A paradigm is the set of beliefs, assumptions, practices, even rituals of a scientific community; it takes in that community's body of knowledge and the means it employs to protect and perpetuate its influence, e.g. systems of training and qualifications, or the institution of 'peer review' in assessing articles submitted to journals. Therefore, nursing belongs to a nursing paradigm that is distinct from the medical paradigm, even though they both share beliefs about an independent world of facts (sometimes referred to as the independent thesis) and that, by and large, we gain knowledge about this independent world via scientific endeavour (sometimes referred to as the knowledge thesis). Child and adolescent nursing has its own paradigm of theory owned by this distinct community within nursing *per se.* This shares theory from child development, social psychology, behaviourism, medicine, and many others. The term paradigm revolution describes the process whereby one paradigm or group of beliefs within a given community is replaced by another. Thus, the classic example that the sun circled the earth belonged to theological science and was overthrown by the rise in experimental philosophy. Copernicus (1473–1543) shattered the static medieval world view by picturing the earth circling the sun. Galileo (d1642) verified this hypothesis using telescopic observation. The original factual beliefs were shattered and became irrelevant to the new. These episodes of revolution can be separated by long periods of 'normal science'.

Nursing today is sometimes referred to as being in a pre-revolutionary paradigm (Fawcett, 1984); that is, we are now in a period in its development in which it is attempting to ascertain its own epistemology and methodology distinct from other disciplines, such as medicine, sociology, and psychology. In reality, it is much more useful to conceive this period as a stage when child and adolescent nursing is finding its feet and utilising theory from other disciplines, including mainstream nursing theory. This process can be seen as consistent with a (M)odernist project, the logical development of efficient specialisms. Advancing nursing practice in this speciality aims to push the boundaries of these theories and discourses. The ill-defined nature of these boundaries reflects the complexity of the numerous theories and models that presently guide child and adolescent nursing practice. In child and adolescent nursing, there seems to be an acceptance that theories and models of nursing, utilised and developed specifically for adults, are equally useful for children and adolescents. Theories such as those of Peplau (1952/1988) and Orem (1991) and those of personality and development are, at present, the best we have to help us, as nurses, structure the care we provide. However, in all its complexity, nursing has to adhere to many compromises, economical forces, and competing theories at any one time. The competing theories that have been dominant for the past thirty years have as their aim, in part, to answer the following questions :

- What is the nature of nursing
- What is the nature of health
- What is the nature of the patient
- What are the effects of the environment?

These questions make up the four facets of the meta-paradigm of nursing (nursing/health/person/environment); a meta-paradigm of nursing that aims to include holism, adaptation, affiliated-individuation and self-care as central tenets to a profession struggling to locate an independent recognition and power/knowledge base.

The meta-paradigm of nursing

The four concepts (person, environment, health, nursing) are those which have been called the 'metaparadigm of nursing' (Fawcett, 1984). It is these four concepts that encapsulate all nursing activities and attempt to provide a boundary between that which is considered nursing and that which is not. Within the boundary, health is seen as a state of physical, mental and social well-being. It is not merely the absence of disease or illness. The concepts are broad and interrelated, but are also considered to be entities in themselves. They are entities that are also the concern of other professional groups apart from nursing (except the concept of nursing itself). Each concept has, to varying degrees, been the central focus of differing nursing models that promote the therapeutic use of self, adaptation, interaction, and behavioural interventions. Without these guiding concepts, nursing ceases to be a profession with a modernist mission. The meta-paradigm of nursing (person, environment, health, nursing) concerns everything we do as nurses. Admissions, assessments, care planning, and discharge planning are just a few of the roles that the average nurse, practising within the remit of child and adolescent mental health, performs. These roles and the many others also belong to the remit of adult, elderly, and community mental health nursing. The concepts are thought to be universal, but our claim to universality questions the underlying foundations of specialism and (M)odernism.

The prospect of a unifying view that every nurse will accept is not achievable. As Fawcett (1989) writes, 'Our sense of unity is an illusion', but she defends the notion of the whole person as being 'an indispensable organising concept'. So nursing continues to attempt to create a complete embracing theory of nursing, a task that is philosophically and theoretically impossible and, as we argue throughout this book, a (M)odernist project doomed to failure. However, as noted by Fawcett (1989), the idea of holism is an organising concept and, as such, is a way to view the four concepts that constitute the meta-paradigm. It is, therefore, argued that the uncertain position in which nursing currently finds itself is linked, in Kuhnian terms, to the pre-revolutionary status of conceptual models of nursing practice. The notion of a meta-paradigm of nursing that is free from the dominant positivist paradigm is a myth, which cannot be hidden by the advancement of holistic practice. Drew (1988) proposed that, in recoiling from the male-dominated, reductionist, disease-orientated medical approach to nursing, science has, perhaps, unintentionally narrowed its scope, primarily to study the social and behavioural sciences. Trnobranski (1993) noted that the move away from cure to care is associated with greater interest in the behavioural and social sciences, such as psychology and sociology. It is argued that, in leaning towards the behavioural and sociological sciences at the expense of the biological, nurse educationalists have developed a philosophy of incomplete holism and, therefore, an incomplete meta-paradigm.

Summary so far ...

We hope that the complex issues discussed so far have not led the reader to feel that none of it makes any sense and is irrelevant to nursing. In short, child and adolescent mental health nursing is now in a Post HAS (1995) period. To date, it has been driven at a theoretical and, to some extent, at a practice level by developments within mainstream psychiatry and child developmental psychology. The philosophical underpinnings of all theory are guided by differing paradigms. These paradigms differ in the way that they view the reality in which we live. For 200 years, the dominant paradigm seen in the age of the Enlightenment has been positivism, which is characterised by a search for grand universal truths. When analysed in terms of the meta-paradigm of nursing, these are truths regarding the nature of man, nursing, the environment, and health. This paradigm remains dominant in nursing in a modern age that is obsessed with a search for certainty, structure, and progress, and is often related to the success of capitalism. However, there is a group of opposing philosophies that can be broadly termed postmodern. These include phenomenology, existentialism, structuralism, post-structuralism, and deconstructionism. These are now discussed to provide a platform for the remainder of the book.

Postmodernist thought

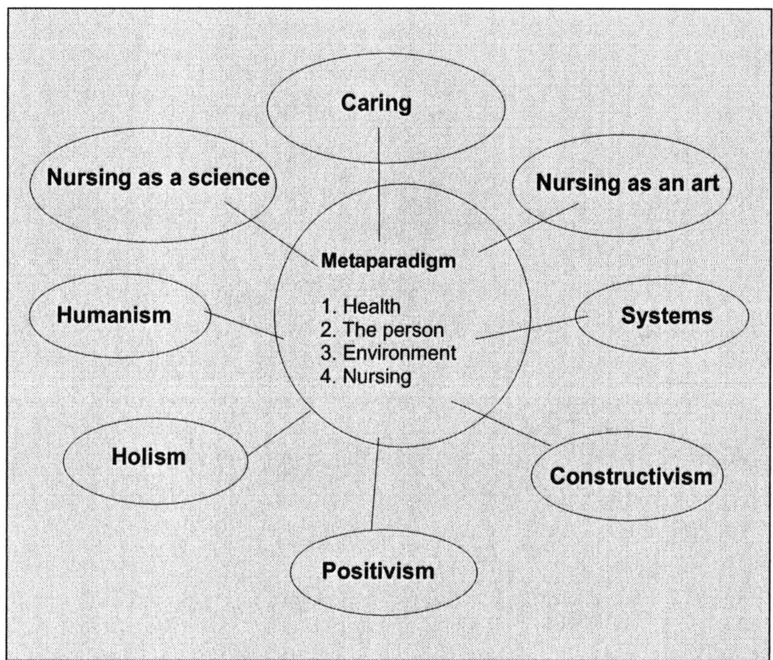

Figure 1.1: Philosophical concepts and the meta-paradigm of nursing

The claim that a meta-paradigm of nursing can give a unifying view that is non-positivist in nature (as argued by Fawcett (1992)) has not been achieved and, in our view, never will be. The philosophical ideas that we discuss now, if nothing else, should emphasise the disunity. As noted by Draper (1993), models of nursing are being advocated and taken as the necessary basis of clinical practice in British nursing, without there having been sufficiently rigorous debate about their empirical foundations, epistemological status, or practical significance. This warns us of the difficulty of deciding what will count as mental health nursing's knowledge base—if we seek to outline a new postmodern meta-paradigm for nursing. However, Onega (1991) highlights several significant philosophical notions that may be shared by all mental health nurses. These are:

1. The nature of human beings;
2. The nature of health;
3. The nature of mental health nursing;
4. The nature of human existence; and

5. The nature of reality.

These five concepts are similar to those proposed by Fawcett's (1989) original meta-paradigm of nursing (environment, person, health, nursing). As a basis for a paradigm of child and adolescent nursing, these concepts allow (possibly within the intellectual tradition of positivism) a tentative platform for analysing the notions of the science and art of nursing, within the holistic approach advocated by the theoretical approaches of constructivism and constructionism. The only difference is the emphasis individual theorists place on each of the concepts. The history of nursing theory is littered with frustrated attempts to achieve a unified theory of nursing science. Such attempts help justify the call for separation into specialisms, such as child and adolescent mental health nursing. When this happens, each specialism takes into account current theory relevant to the said specialism. Such current critical theory has to take into account the critical theories of the twentieth century, which will now be briefly outlined because of their importance throughout the remainder of the book. They are:

- Modernism
- Phenomenology
- Structuralism
- Post-structuralism
- Post-modernism.

Modernism

As with post-modernism, (M)odernism is extremely hard to define. It is about technological rationality, 'progress', and the harnessing of nature by man. Modernism is often viewed as man coming of age, when humanity was able to understand itself and the environment through the process of scientific endeavour. It is often identified as beginning with Descartes, the Enlightenment and the 'age of reason'. For others, it is the industrial revolutions and the rise of empiricism in Britain; for nursing, the mid twentieth century with the advent of the nursing process and models, and a growing professional role. The question of modernism in child and adolescent mental health nursing is also a child of the sudden onslaught of modernisation. This primarily relates to the effects of positivist scientific methodologies and the forceful metaphysical epistemologies belonging to the traditions of Western philosophical thought. Modern nursing, therefore, reflects the conditions of this conceptual age of man finally mastering nature. There is, at the core of contemporary nursing, the belief in meta-paradigms, holism, humanism and other concepts as shown in *Figure 1.1*. This organising and professionalising is what it is to be modern—to live in a man-made reality. The modern conditions of nursing, as exposed by paradigms, meta-paradigms, and models, have engendered a new response in that modern preoccupation with the individual; that the individual child who, when being nursed, has a name, a life history, and a care plan. The child is surrounded by modernity of nursing, which, itself, is still in its infancy and in need of much correction.

Postmodernism

It is important to spend a considerable amount of time exploring the nature of what modernism is and how it is utilised in this book. Our premise is that post-modernism is necessarily related to the conditions of late capitalism. It goes beyond a descriptive understanding of nursing that simply classifies it according to differences between each speciality, to analyse the conditions that have given rise to it. Nursing can be seen to constitute the epiphenomena of broader underlying social forces. An understanding of such, therefore, opens up the possibilities of how nursing might be understood beyond the narrow focus of traditional nursing discourse. Post-modernist thought can be viewed as a grouping of critique that, to varying degrees, all present facets of a similar philosophy. The major tenets of such thoughts centre on a particular range of methodologies—a set of tools—for addressing nursing in terms of a wider cultural context. Exploring the concepts and judgements that we as nurses make regarding the care of young people is to begin examining the discourses belonging to the wider cultural context. However, that examination does not seek to provide an all embracing unified view or nursing knowledge as attempted by many nursing theorists previously described. Postmodernism in nursing comprises a complex set of reactions to modern philosophy, such as phenomenology, humanism, holism, and structural thought, to re-emphasise *reactions*, rather than any agreement on substantive doctrines. As noted by McInerny (1995: 634), postmodern philosophy typically opposes foundationalism, essentialism, and realism. The presuppositions to be set aside are very deep assumptions shared by the leading sixteenth, seventeenth, and eighteenth century philosophers. For Nietzsche, Heidegger, Foucault, and Jacques Derrida, the presuppositions to be set aside are as old as metaphysics, and are best exemplified by Plato (McInerny, 1995: 634). So, in the spirit of postmodernism, we argue the need to call into question the way we, as nurses caring for the mentally health of children and young people, view the everyday concepts, language and value judgements of everyday practice.

As such, according to McInery (1995: 634) postmodern philosophy is usefully regarded as a complex cluster concept. It has an anti or post epistemological standpoint, which rejects the claim that our temporary human systems of knowledge and 'truth' can be accurate representations of reality. It rejects final vocabularies, principles, categories, meta-narratives and, as proposed by McInery (1995: 634), 'the traditional dream of a complete, unique and closed explanatory system typically fuelled by binary oppositions'. In addition, postmodernism makes strong play of individual experience being subject to gender, culture and ethnicity, so making possible a strong alliance with nursing. Postmodernism in nursing rejects the totalising tendency of metaphysics, foundationalism, and universalising of mainstream thought, which includes positivism, holism, and humanism. The postmodernist nurse is suspicious of any grand meta theories, including those traditional views of subjectivity and history in child development. The examples are numerous, including the views we hold about theories of psycho-sexual development, cognitive testing and the onset of illness.

In their preface, Pasquali *et al* (1989) consider the implications of these philosophical approaches to mental health nursing. They argue that no one theory or conceptual model can provide a complete basis for understanding all aspects of human functioning, or the complexities of human behaviour. The question is whether such theories can assist the child mental health nurse in providing the most advanced care to children and younger people. These theories have to take into account the philosophical assumptions about man, health, nursing, and the environment, which are part of the total paradigm. These include Freudian and Rogerian theories of self and, particularly in the case of child and adolescent mental health, the theories of Klien and Erikson, all of which can be viewed as 'modern' in the sense we wish to oppose. It is also usual to make specific reference to behaviourism within child development. From this collection of incompatible and opposing theories, nursing scholars have postulated hypotheses and formulated questions to create conceptual models of nursing practice. To do this, they have taken concepts from various paradigms of thought, particularly sociology, medicine and psychology. The most popular recipes in mental health begin with Peplau (1952/1988). It is assumed that nursing is naturally a people-orientated process that has finally shed its dependence upon the biological mechanism of medicine. (Of course, there are times when people are biologically unwell, so it would be unwise to neglect the advances medicine has made in healing people with technology, and stick rigidly to the humanist, holistic systems approach advocated by certain mental health books and journals). However, it is worth bearing in mind that the authors feel medicine is not the same as psychiatry. The latter is a particular strand of medicine that is also struggling to maintain a unified view of mental health, which is posited on the diagnosis and mostly biological classification of groups of symptoms. Psychiatry is, in origin, a positivist creation and one that advanced nursing practice finds alien due to its dependence upon logical, reductionist formulations of childhood and adolescence. This will become more clear in the next section that discusses the art of nursing—that which distinguishes nursing—as a unique profession. For now, it is necessary to highlight the main branches of twentieth century thought already known and utilised in the conceptual foundations of nursing.

Phenomenology

Questions of phenomenology address humankind's 'situatedness' in the world, and focus on the 'depthlessness' of modern existence. Phenomenology offers a model that is philosophically subjectivist and anti-positivist, and praised in nursing science and art. Phenomenology is often linked to humanism and existentialism (particularly in the work of RD Laing) in a type of constructivist mish-mash. It is seen as a foundation for the exploration of the 'subjective self'. As a model, it probes below the surfaces of individual existence and enquires about the fundamental basis of the human condition. It is precisely by exposing the impoverished mechanisms by which nursing has traditionally had theory imposed on it, that phenomenology attempts to point the way forward to an approach to nursing knowledge that seeks to transcend the limitations of technological modernism and positivism. However, phenomenology is itself a modern attempt to understand the abstract puzzles of what it means to be human. It offers a philosophical approach that is becoming popular with nurses, whereby they are licensed to explore the individuality and uniqueness of young people's experiences. They can, therefore, offer a modern counter-balance to the existing nursing epistemology that is left behind in the realms of the 'age of reason'.

Structuralism

Structuralism through the study of semiology and language offers a flexible, contemporary model for understanding nursing knowledge and practice. It indicates how nursing can be understood in terms of the language, culture and power it utilises. In doing so, it opens up a domain often not fully appreciated by nurses, or overlooked entirely. Indeed, nursing has tended to stress the functional aspects of practice to the detriment of the structural dimension. The question of how nursing might be re-defined semantically is further elaborated by the post-structuralist contributions.

Post-structuralism

The post-structuralist contribution to modern critical analysis shifts increasingly away from a discussion of existence towards one of content. Indeed, in the work of Michel Foucault (1971), the authority of medicine is called into question. Post-structuralist work serves as a necessary correction to the often inflated claims ascribed to medicine and nursing by health care professionals themselves.

Last remarks

This chapter has aimed to provide a starting point for exploring the philosophical issues relevant to nursing mentally ill children and young people. It has touched upon a number of very complex, but significant concepts. These include those which are relevant in the domain of a unified nursing knowledge base, namely, paradigm, meta-paradigm, positivism, constructivist/constructionist paradigm, and holism. Philosophy may seem confusing and perhaps irrelevant to actual nursing practice, but we tried to suggest that a careful critical analysis of theoretical assumptions can show why aspects of daily practice are going wrong. Such an exploration of nursing issues highlights the questioning of long held assumptions about the role of nursing ill children within the traditional positivistic paradigm. (M)odernism has been viewed as the use of the characteristic methods of a discipline to criticise the discipline itself (Greenberg, 1980), as he says, not in order to subvert it, but to entrench it more firmly in its area of competence. The self criticism of (M)odernism grows out of, but is not the same thing as the criticism of the Enlightenment. As noted by Greenberg (1980), the Enlightenment criticises from outside (the way criticism in its usually accepted sense does); (M)odernism criticises from the inside through the procedures, themselves, of the activity that is being criticised. Hence, the anti-positivistic epistemology of (M)odernist critique. This chapter has highlighted the scientific paradigms of thought in nursing and the opposing forces of holism and caring, which are seen as being a process belonging to nursing practice within the dynamics of most nurse-child relationships. Moreover, holism and caring, properly understood, are the cornerstones of nursing's proper contribution to health care. It is hoped that this chapter has highlighted the ambiguous space in which modern nursing is beginning to find itself as it struggles, not as a whole, but as individual practitioners and small collective specialities, to locate itself within the plethora of competing epistemologies and theoretical positions. (M)odernism as a critique allows for this struggle to be illuminated and addressed, be it from a phenomenological or structural perspective. Indeed, Modernism allows these to be self critical.

A further premise of this chapter has been concerned with the struggle of epistemological location by virtue of attempting to identify the tenets that ascribe uniqueness to nursing *per se*. What modernism has allowed is a critique of how nursing defines itself; that is, its own particular essence. We saw that the meta-paradigm of nursing identifies the four distinct domains of person, environment, health, and nursing as the significant concerns, but this is presented from within the typical positivistic framework that one has come to expect from a profession struggling to create a viable epistemology. A (M)odernist critique of such a position emphasises that each nursing speciality has to be non-assimilated, that is, each has to demonstrate that the experiences they provide, both theoretically and at a practice level, are valuable in their own right and not to be obtained by any other kind of activity. Therefore, child and adolescent mental health nursing needs science and art, an epistemology and ontology that are inseparable and reducible to the sum of their parts, and able to demonstrate its uniqueness on its own account. In this period of nursing after the Health Advisory Service Report (1995), the nursing care of young people has to be distinguished from other types of nursing. It has to be determined by operations peculiar to itself. By doing so, it narrows its sphere of competence, but makes its possession of this area all the more secure theoretically as well as in name. This is not a surprising discovery as most nurses practising within this speciality would agree. However, as argued throughout this chapter, a broader analysis and deconstruction of the typical concepts, language, and value judgements of what we do, as we go about nursing mentally ill children and adolescents, presents itself as a modernist analysis and a Postmodernist critique, utilising the philosophical tenets proposed by phenomenology, structuralism, and post-structuralism.

This chapter has also argued the premise that child and adolescent mental health nursing, like other specialities, has a unique and proper area of competence that coincides with the unique nature of its medium: children and young people. Once again, this may appear not too surprising, but it is an important consideration when we consider the generic nature of the theory we use to construct our beliefs and assumptions regarding mental illness and the concepts of child development. Is child and adolescent mental health nursing pure? What are the limitations? Are they the same as those dictated by the positivist tradition?

Chapter 2
The art and science of nursing: the holistic paradox

'The individual self becomes a medium for the culture and its language'
Parker *et al* (1995: 36)

Dialogue:

Dean: Is nursing a science, or is it an art?

Sandy: Oh, surely this is a debate that will continue forever?

Dean: But the trouble is, it doesn't offer any pragmatic stuff that's any use in practice, does it?

Sandy: No, but it offers a starting point from which the knowledge base of nursing can be explored.

Dean: But that doesn't help does it? I mean it seems to me that every other word spoken in nursing at the moment is a buzz word, such as holism, humanism or systems. We speak of them as though they're really useful when we're all just trying to be trendy.

Sandy: I don't think so...it's far better to be concerned with holism than reduce everything down into a diagnosis or biological cause isn't it?

Dean: Arh...but is that what we really do?

Sandy: I think so...I mean nurses take into account the social, psychological, and physical aspects of a child's welfare in order to care for them holistically, don't they? And its usually done in a humanist way.

Dean: I'm not so sure. I think there are two distinct point here. Firstly, the holism one and, secondly, the idea that we all practice in a type of Rogerian or eclectic humanist way so as to promote the art of nursing. We do it because we're conditioned.

Sandy: Yeah, so?

Dean: Well, I think what we say we do is not the same as what we do, is it? Both holism and humanism are philosophies that work very well in this modern age. They've given nursing a new lease of life. You know, a chance to have nursing philosophies develop a role, while at the same time remaining subversive to positivism.

Sandy: Just because you're sceptical doesn't mean they'll go away. We still need to re-think them, don't we?

Dean: I'm not sceptical, I just think that nursing owes it to itself to be sceptical you know... perhaps any philosophy is better than no philosophy at all, but surely not one that maintains the *status quo* in nursing's subversive position.

Sandy: Sometimes I don't believe all the parts of you!

Theses for this chapter

- ❑ The philosophy of humanism, holism and systems philosophy are seen as fundamental for the scientific and artistic delivery of nursing theory.

Background and aims

Writers at the beginning of the nineteenth century argued that people bring meaning into existence through their spiritual life, which is exemplified, at least in part, by the arts (Smith, 1997: 338). That romanticism and its attempt to promote a shared culture echoes the lack of integration between the science and art of nursing. Much controversy and academic argument rages regarding both the art and the science of nursing. Each are seen as being distinctly separate concepts—there is no holistic knowledge base. The idea that the art of nursing is about the actual delivery of practice, that is, the therapeutic relationship with its dependence on phenomenological and humanistic subjectivity of the young person, is so often shown as being opposed to the objectivity of science. The aim of this chapter is not to add to the futility of this debate, but rather to offer an introduction to the issue to the bemused reader, and to discuss the philosophical nature of holism in relation to modern nursing.

1. To explore the concepts of art and science in relation to the body of nursing knowledge; and
2. To take up the previous chapter's discussion of twentieth century critical thought, in particular, the relevance of holism and system theory.

Introduction

The positivist and post-scientific paradigms have an empirical epistemology, based on a corresponding theory of truth and a commitment to quantitative methods. Critical theory and constructivist stances derive from a subjectivist epistemology and a reliance on qualitative methods. Nursing does not sit comfortably in either camp, but, generally, can be seen as anti-positivist (Playle, 1995). Therefore, there is much debate regarding the nursing as a science *vs* nursing as an art argument, which reflects the wider debate regarding the scientific paradigms discussed in the previous chapter. The possible demise of positivism in nursing reflects the growing belief in holism rather than reductionism. In positivism, problems with the verification of hypotheses (logical positivism) led Popper (1959) to propose the more rigorous requirement of falsification of hypotheses (this has led to the expansion of several schools of thought, including critical rationalism/conventionalism/post-positivism). The abandonment of certainties of positivism left the philosophy of science on a slippery slope towards a position where choice between theories appeared to be more than a matter of taste (post modernism) (Hollinger, 1994). In nursing, this taste has been predominantly in the guise of constructivist and constructionist approaches. These focus on the understanding of actions and meanings of individuals, are founded on understandings of what exists, and this is dependent upon what individuals perceive to exist. Thus, it is its ontological claim that most differentiates constructivism from the other philosophies of science, such as positivism. However, the powers of social structures (constructionism) cannot be reduced to those of individuals. Thus 'explanations of the actions of individuals often requires not a micro (reductionist) appeal to their inner constitution (though that may be relevant too), but a macro appeal to the social structures in which they are located. This highlights the epistemological difference between constructivism and constructionism. The former is located within the phenomenological/existential tradition of philosophy, while the latter is considered postmodern and post-structuralist.

Exploring the concepts of art and science

We have tried to show that, in general, nursing is saturated by many theoretical and philosophical doctrines that can be loosely considered modernist, not only due to their continued existence and considered importance in twentieth century nursing, but because of their emphatic claims to logic, truth and objectivity. The identification of paradigms and meta-paradigms places nursing firmly in the scientific domain, and child and adolescent nursing as a sub-set within it. Therefore, to be modern can now be seen as a battlefield using weapons and tactics shaped and legitimised by ideological doctrines. One of the many premises of this book is that nursing is a (M)odern phenomenon; until recently, much of its self analysis has taken place within positivist technological assumptions, as opposed to those considered postmodern. Our task, although it feels strange at times, is actually to question the validity of the positivist world view. The positivist world seems to present its own meta-paradigms as a natural state of reality, when, in fact, nursing and all of its contemporary modernism is really no more than a man-made (medicine/nurse-made) phenomenon. The many philosophies, including holism, humanism, and phenomenology, merely serve to prolong the positivist era and, by their existence, provide evidence that nursing is (M)odernist and belongs to a twentieth century that has the illusion of having conquered nature, and is attempting to finish off the conquest of reality as we know it. The central issue of art and science is ultimately a concern of nursing because it reflects the futile, but widespread demand (within many parts of society) to do away with uncertainty.

As noted by Appleton (1993), 'documented historical views and contemporary theory supports the belief that nursing is a science and an art'. The science is understood to be the positivist, rational, and a universal part of a nursing knowledge base. It is seen as the pure and applied science that is usually evaluated in terms of methodological discussion. The debate regarding methodologies and nursing's knowledge base serves to identify the underlying paradigmatic tenets of practice, that is, scientifically researched practice, which is concerned with the natural and social sciences. This, according to Cushing (1994), manifests itself in arguments relating to qualitative and quantitative paradigms of inquiry that prevent nursing becoming something more than an applied science. By concentrating on methodological interests, there is a tendency to neglect the contribution of the theoretical achievements nursing is capable of in terms of an epistemological nature. Such theory includes the meta-paradigmatic work of Fawcett (1989), Peplau (1952/1988) and other nurse theorists. According to Timpson (1996), this reflects the fact that nursing theory remains poorly evaluated, articulated, or understood and in a dilemma regarding 'a lack of direction' (Packard and Polifroni, 1991). The inability of nursing to provide unified conceptual models and a complete scientific knowledge base reflects, for many nurses, the limitation of scientific theoretical inquiry, full stop. As noted by Benner and Wrubel (1989), the majority of contemporary nursing theories can be located within the classical scientific mode, which directs methodology towards the experimental science paradigm. The discipline of child and adolescent mental health nursing, and nursing generally, may be evaluated by the identification and clarification of the body of knowledge that is considered *unique* to nursing (Timpson, 1996). A discipline of nursing, therefore, is more than just a science. It is, as noted by Gray and Pratt (1991, cited in Timpson, 1996), 'a professional discipline having a concern for human health and well being, a blending of science and art'.

The art of nursing is unique to nursing, the science is not. A definition of the art of nursing would have to include, firstly, a metaphysical notion of 'being' and 'doing' practice; and, secondly, there would have to be notions of humanist/interpersonal use of self and caring that are seen as being peculiar to nursing. It is these facets of self and caring that are seen to separate nursing from all other health care disciplines. However, a friendly critic (Pursey) might ask, how do we record, account for, train for, respect and dignify these facets of nursing ? In a sense, do we not presuppose (often automatically) their presence in a person making a career choice? Or do they have a status like those polite legal fictions, that (for example) soldiers are courageous, officers 'gallant gentlemen' and lawyers 'learned'? (These issue of caring and humanism will be discussed in the next chapter). Thirdly, the concepts of holism, nursing as a process, constructionism, and phenomenology are seen as postmodern and a break from positivism. Postmodern, because nursing as an art accepts the individuality of humans and attempts, in practice, to disregard the universality of prestigious and, ostensibly, deductive academic doctrines (Fawcett and Downs, 1992). The attempt of nursing scholars to reconcile the epistemological differences between positivism and anti-positivist doctrines has deflected concern away from the fact that nursing has particular and special ontological concerns, which are central to its actual practice, more so than any other health care profession. These ontological concerns are the subjective and non-universal experiences of patients whose experiences nurses, as carers, are more likely to be aware of than other professionals who perform specific tasks, such as duties, and then leave. The art of nursing is concerned with the individual and the interpersonal contact between nurse and child/patient. Hence, we can understand the concern with interpersonal dimensions of practice found in mental health models of care.

We want to claim that nursing has within its grasp the ability to contribute uniquely to health care by enlarging its own art, thus expanding its knowledge base as a distinct discipline. In order to do this, it has to be prepared to make some breaks with its current dependency on the biomedical/physical model of nursing science, and instead acknowledge more fully the importance of interpersonal (constructivist and constructionist) relations in providing a form of practice unique to nursing. The same is true for child and adolescent nursing, which needs to create its own knowledge base apart from the adult speciality and the medical paradigms of science.

The advance of phenomenology and hermeneutics in the qualitative tradition of anthropology and ethnography in nursing has helped in this evaluation of nursing epistemology, as noted by Timpson (1996). It also heads the advancement of the art of nursing as a unique activity in health care provision. As noted by Cushing (1994), phenomenology is popular among nurses because it accords well with clinical concerns. Such relevance to nursing is highlighted in comments made by Ray (1990; 1991). Morse (1989) raises questions about nursing borrowing other disciplines' theoretical assumptions and about the application of research methodologies, but, despite these concerns and as noted by Cushing (1994), phenomenology is treated with apparent respect by many nursing scholars. It permits practice to be more individually orientated as a *care* process and, as such, more readily makes the individual reflection, and humanist and holistic approaches, applicable to ordinary practice. It assumes that reality can be perceived and understood subjectively by each individual for him/herself. Phenomenology is, therefore, viable and useful in practice. Theoretically, its opponents criticise its lack of empiricism, so its epistemology remains tenuous, but its methodology continues to be enthusiastically endorsed by nursing scholars. The art of nursing when combined with its science provides a knowledge base that is encompassed within the holist meta-paradigm of nursing.

If we agree that a nursing knowledge base contains those concepts of a meta-paradigm, proposed by Fawcett (1989), and an ongoing debate regarding the science and art of nursing that is guided by the philosophical motivation of holism and humanism, it becomes clear that nursing mentally ill children and young people is firmly based within the same ambiguous space. It is clear that nursing is not a series of tasks, views, and opinions detached from theoretical and philosophical underpinnings, even though textbooks still give the impression that a coherent whole will somehow appear from a mere list of components.

Science		Art	
Fact	Universality	Individuality	Opinion
Value-free	Positivist	Constructivist (tionist)	Value-laden
Curing	Reductionism	Holism	Caring
Masculine	Structure/ Outcome	Process	Feminine
Clarity	Rational	Intuitive	Muddle
Technical	Certainty	Knowing/ Exploring	Random
Empirical	Logic	Heuristics	Phenomenological

Figure 2.1: Concepts usually associated with an over-emphatic separation of art and science

A delicate balance

The nature of caring in nursing mentally ill young people and children brings with it important issues of mothering, attachment, containment, family processes, and the necessity to nurture and understand the nurse-patient relationship, which is often experienced as being more demanding than that in adult nursing. This is not to doubt that each speciality has its own peculiar kind of experience. Thus, the application of knowledge and skill to bring about a desired result encompasses, at a theoretical level, issues of nursing science. For example, the need to ensure physical developmental milestones have been reached, the careful monitoring of social interactions that are often taken for granted in adult nursing and, most difficult perhaps, the need to understand the complex psychological fantasies and methods of expression that children and young people utilise in a world that appears very large for them. Development in childhood often means that abstract thought should make use of more creative nursing techniques and more rigid time structuring. At a practical level, the art of nursing tries to make the best use of its scientific knowledge base as a process. For example, a young person may not be able to comprehend that he/she is scared and angry due to past events in his/her life (this is an assumption), but the nurse will be able to utilise such knowledge to help the child express him/herself. The ability to guide, support, and make the best use of humanistic approaches to create growth is the core of the art of nursing. The nursing scholar, Rogers (1970), contends that nursing is both a science and a humanistic art. The idea that, in the absence of any certain knowledge, nursing should hedge its bets and always be practised as a science and an art reflects its uncertainty as a youthful profession, but nursing is a practice-based profession that needs to acknowledge the importance of both. Similarly, the nursing scholar, Parse (1981), reflects the existential phenomenological writings of Martin Heidegger (1962), Jean Paul Sartre (1992) and Maurice Merleau-Ponty (1948), which promote constructivist metaphysical assertions that subjectivity is the starting point for all our knowledge of what exists in the world. Therefore, the world of the child can be seen to be very different in terms of the individual constructs developing minds create. This can never be scientifically measured and is best explored via the art of nursing. The chief British contributor to nursing theory, Roper (1988), supports the view that nursing is both a science and an art, and calls nursing a therapeutic intervention in itself, that is, an intervention which is holist. Therefore, holism is something that appears central in modern nursing and gives us a philosophy, which attempts to view the patient as an active and unique being, incorporating social, biological and psychological systems. An exploration of holism the champion of (M)odernist nursing will now be given.

Summary so far...

Postmodernism can be viewed as an approach to critical analysis that questions both the theory and practice of modern child and adolescent nursing. It comes in various guises and is a product of (M)odernism itself. It could be argued that its existence is possible only at the end of the twentieth century. Instead of attempting to produce universal truths, postmodernist critique does the opposite. Firstly, it questions the very metaphysics that are at the foundations of positivism and, secondly, it illuminates the discourses related to power that guide human history. Holism is seen as the major achievement of nursing in the second half of the twentieth century. It is a symptom of the twentieth century, and fundamentally anti-positivist. It is often viewed as an opposite to reductionism. Usually, it is typically considered to promote an understanding of personhood as a collection of inter-related systems (physical, psychological, social, spiritual, and environmental). This is reflected in many nursing models and contemporary journal articles. It is related to issues of coincidence, cause and effect, time and space, in that the whole universe is seen as inter-connected.

Holism

The American Holistic Nurses Association (1992) defines holism as follows:

> *'The concept of wellness: that state of harmony between mind, body, emotions and spirit in an ever changing environment.'*

The holistic health movement encompasses many divergent philosophies, religious doctrines and psychological theories (Stensrud, 1984; cited in Kolcaba, 1997). As noted by Kolcaba (1997), metaphysical holism is the view that reality is comprised of wholes. As such, the philosophical issue of holism has appeared, traditionally, within the paradigms of biology, psychology, and the human sciences. Hence, the attraction to nursing and postmodernist philosophy. Metaphysically speaking, holism holds that the whole has some properties that its parts lack. These cannot necessarily be seen (as in the case of the atom) and there is a denial of deductibility, whereas affirming the deductibility as in reductionism can also be termed methodological individualism. As noted by Addis (1995: 336), in the philosophy of the social sciences, where 'holism' has had its most common use in philosophy, the many issues have been reduced to that of these two: metaphysical holism *vs* methodological individualism. This terminology reflected the positivist criticism that holism goes beyond empirical facts in postulating social wholes and identifying the reality of society beyond individual persons (as in constructionist theory). Individualism, however, is supposed to be empirical or at least more so for the purpose of describing and explaining social phenomena. For nursing, with its many claims of holistic practice, these philosophical issues are rarely if ever discussed. It is just assumed that holism is a good thing because it considers the 'whole child or young person' within the realms of what is happening for them in their physical, psychological, and social experiences. As such, nursing is concerned with issues of both metaphysical and methodological holism. However, this comfortable acceptance does not illuminate the inconsistency between the two philosophical strands of holism. For example, Jan Smuts (1926) originally argued for a holism in which the universe evolved towards producing wholes within a hierarchy based on degrees of complexity. Without being able to be tested, holism has been developed by general systems theorists, such as von Bertalanffy (1968), who suggested that a hierarchical ordering of nested systems comprises reality as a whole. What all this means for nursing is that holism first has metaphysical and empirical underpinnings, which are not necessarily compatible (highlighting its incompleteness) and, second, its use as a guiding philosophy within the meta-paradigm of nursing is not necessarily straightforward. In order to try and explore this further, Kolcaba's (1997) model of three types of whole offers a useful instrument with which to look more closely at a supposedly simple philosophy.

Three types of whole

According to Kolcaba (1997), within the life sciences, taxonomies have grown up around systems, organisms and persons. These three concepts provide a way of exploring the philosophy of holism. Within these three, there are the two core concepts of 'whole' and 'part'. A whole is made up of parts, thus everything can be either viewed as a part or as a whole. This, according to Kolcaba, is the whole/part dichotomy. It is the most obvious phenomenon that practising nurses relate to within the practice area. For example, when a young person is admitted to a Tier 4 provision, it is usual for a nursing assessment to consider more than just the major symptoms that led to the admission in the first place. The young person can be viewed as being depressed, but the depression can be seen as being just part of his or her social circumstances and so on. Therefore, holism has within it notions of boundaries similar to the paradigm of nursing with its four major concepts of person, health, environment, and nursing.

The concept of system

As noted by Kolcaba (1997), a system can be defined as a group of interrelated parts that jointly perform function (see *Figure 2.2*). The concept of **function**, because the word implies some kind of performance, indicates the range of parts comprising the system. The system consists of what is required for the function to be performed. The per-

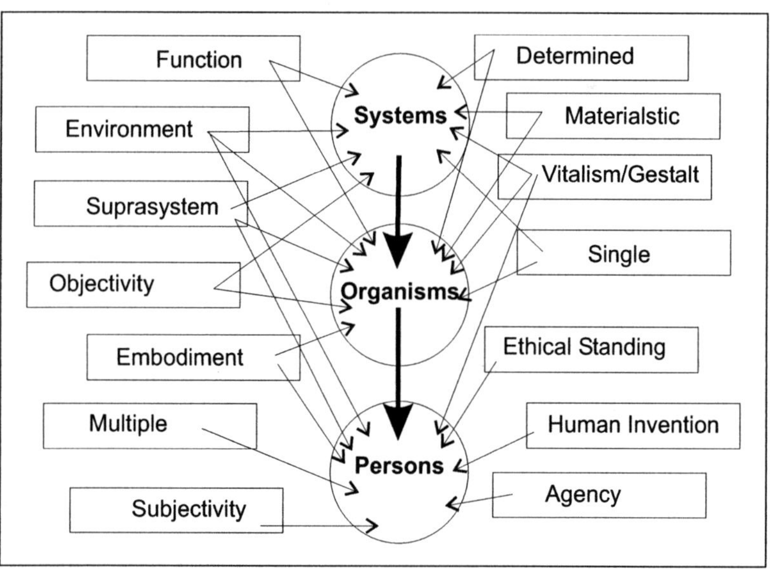

Figure 2.2: Conceptualising holism

formance of function is the measure for health of the system. If the elements of a system are decided by function then parts of systems are also aspects of the environment. Whole systems fall short of a whole organism. From the point of view of the concept of a system, the concept of organism as a super-system is little more than a metaphor. The concept of an organism, unlike the concept of a system, involves the organism's distinction from the environment. Separation from the environment allows for an intelligible notion of the individual. The metaphysics underlying biological science is essentially materialistic. In the general sense, a person is a self or agent which owns a body. If the mind/body identity theory is correct, then ownership of the body would mean ownership of the self. If a dualistic view is correct (Descartes/Peplau) then ownership of the body does not necessarily mean ownership of the soul/mind.

The art of nursing does not produce falsifiable hypotheses in the way 'good' scientific theory is supposed to do. Every aspect of the art of nursing is a perspective related to a particular view of reality. Yet it would be wrong to deny to art all claims of achieving truth within systems of experience. The art of nursing makes valuable contributions to our understanding of systems and of the world of man. The sociologist can only feel uneasy about any too radical separation of art and science. For after all, the world view of a generation of nurses—or, more exactly, of any group that is historically and sociologically self-contained—is an indivisible whole. Attempts to demarcate the different fields in which the world view manifests itself might be very promising and comfortable from the epistemological point of view, but to the sociologist they appear as violent dissections of the reality he studies. For post-modern nursing philosophy, biology, science, and custom are all aspects of one unitary attitude to reality.

General systems theory

General systems theory has its philosophical origins in a belief in cause and effect, in the view that reality is in a constant state of flux, and in holism. Nursing's emphasis on a whole person orientation stems from its tradition as humanistic practice, that is, the treatment of humanity as a basic principle. As such, humanist philosophy shares the systems belief that man is at the centre of his world, which is interconnected to his complex intra-personal, interpersonal interactions and those with the environment. There is no prime mover as man has agency to create his own being and destiny. However, the systems of which he is part act as forces that cannot be ignored, as they are intrinsic to his being. As an emerging research science, nursing utilises these theories, but tensions among the various holisms of persons, systems, and organisms make it unclear if nursing will follow in the wake of other sciences or pose a new synthesis. Such a new synthesis will have to accommodate the assumption that sets of holisms (sub-sets) create systems and they, in turn, overlap with other systems.

The holist debate is synonymous with discussions of systems, as noted as early as 1965 by Miller (p28): 'systems exist as a synthesis of their parts so that 'the whole is greater than the sum of its parts'. Each system then forms part of a bigger super system so that you can continually search for 'includedness''. Flow of information is a central concept in systems theory and in therapy is utilised in the form of feedback. As early as 1967, Buckley identified three types of information. These are external information of data outside of the system, historical information, and internal information. These types of information enable the system to maintain itself over periods of time and adapt to environmental conditions. As such, systems theory allows the conceptualisation of units and the study of dynamics between subsystems. The culture of a family, Tier 4 adolescent unit and nurses on a particular shift or team can be viewed as a series of systems all flowing to maintain the homeostasis. Generally, adolescent unit cultures are said to be closed, in that they are self-contained as opposed to open systems, which are actively engaging with other environmental systems.

These three dominant theories (systems/organisms/persons), which inform the majority of health care for children and young people, form part of the nursing ideology that structures the care nurses provide. They are interwoven into the nursing cultures, rituals and general assumptions that **the care given is the care needed**. As such, every nurse in community teams and residential units will be in ideological debate about the best nursing practice available on a daily basis, given the resources at hand. The type of working culture helps determine the choice of theoretical models and, in turn, culture is shaped by the ideology that encompasses the styles of leadership teams adopt in order to manage their daily interface and demands. (As such, this raises the impact ideology has on the way we, as nurses, practice. A discussion on nursing ideology is important and is discussed in the following chapters).

'Persons are a human invention in the sense that their self-concept and understanding are products of theirs or other persons' (Kolcaba, 1997). Persons live by rational knowledge and critical judgement under a self concept and world view. The status of personhood is said to entitle the individual to respect as a person, as well as just treatment. The ethical standing of persons also entails responsibilities and obligations to self, others and, as some argue, to the environment. The concepts of systems and organisms are devoid of ethical content. They do not entail agency, that is, the ability to make choices, albeit small ones. The whole-person holist contends that the systemic holist is unduly concerned with body mechanics and that the organismic holist is too narrowly focussed on organismic aetiology and natural history. Persons become ill, not systems. Persons feel ill; organisms behave in an ill manner. Properties of organisms and parts of systems are subordinate to this phenomena.

The trouble with whole-person holism is that selves have experiential parts. While philosophical and psychological theories of personality relate lived experiences to whole person outcomes, desired therapeutic results based on these theories are highly limited. Thus, a holism of persons is far too incomplete to ground a science, let alone an experimental science of health recovery and maintenance. A super-holism comprised of a synthesis of the three is not possible, but what we can do is to use the whole-person holism as a basis for deciding how to treat the other two holisms.

The most striking aspect of Person-based Holism as an organising concept is that persons are subjects that produce, and are products of, subjective experience. They are unlike systems and organisms that are definable by their properties. In a very influential argument, Kant (1785/1956) contended that 'persons are not to be used merely as means to serve our purposes, but that persons are first and always ends in themselves'. The problematical dimension of PBH lies within the contrasting metaphysics of the three holisms. Each implies a faulty reduction. The result of applying systems theory is the reducing of persons to systems—the whole-person holism implies a reduction of large systems in the world—and organisms to persons, subscribing to biological materialism. But persons do not extend into the realms of the environment and natural history. Researchers employing metaphysics use metaphor to mask the stark problems of a faulty reductionism.

Conclusion

It may be thought that systems theory and holism have their chief importance in the health care setting. This appears to be a natural assumption to make considering the daily exposure we, as nurses, have to them. However, as this chapter has highlighted, the philosophical ideas that permeate health care are also all around in the culture we call society. The development of nuclear missile stations, large city planning, and underground railway services all utilise systems and holistic philosophy. We live in an era of technological systems in which systems are used to make sense of, and priorities that are considered useful or profitable. The advent of computer technology and its subsequent language has forced on society its own deep assumptions that everything can be reduced to (or contained within) a simple, technocratic model of cause and effect. This chapter has questioned the perceived pure holism and placed it firmly within the culture and language-dependent society in which it exists. As such, it has been taken out of its typical nursing environment. A little strange perhaps, but it can do no harm to reflect upon one of the philosophical ideas most referred to by theorists of nursing today.

Chapter 3
Child-centred caring

"Without the direction provided by ontological nursing knowledge, the end result of our efforts at inquiry would be chaos..."

(Kikuchi and Simmons, 1992 :35; cited in Brykczynska, 1995: 122)

Dialogue

Dean: We've got to explore the issue of caring because, as a concept, it's very significant.

Sandy: What do you mean?

Dean: Nursing in the modernist sense is concerned with all the technologies and structures that have consequences for the way we view reality, perhaps without even knowing they exist. The concept of caring forms part of these structures. Supposedly it's this 'caring' that distinguishes nursing from all other disciplines.

Sandy: It sounds a bit like a riddle to me. I thought, surely caring is something nurses can take for granted. Isn't it just the result of doing our nursing science in the right way, as responsible human beings?

Dean: It may be, but do we know what the concept of caring really is? Why do we assume that, by demonstrating unconditional positive regard, we are good humanists, for example? I mean, the modern was about newness; the advent of humanist models of care ushered in a vision of Utopia in which technology, systematising, and relationship models heralded a belief that humanism was all that nursing sought. I think the fact remains that humanism is often seen as the art of nursing in practice. The nurse-young person relationship is seen as something universally good. When we look through postmodern glasses, we see that such universals contradict the essence of humanism in practice. How can this be so?

Sandy: I think you're taking this a bit too far.

Dean: The fact is that we believe that the therapeutic use of self is our best tool to care for young people, don't we? The medic puts his faith in science and technology. Humanism is our technology.

Sandy: So?

Dean: Well, I think it's important to explore this a little, because I think we do what we do as nurses by way of relationship-forming and so on, because otherwise there wouldn't be a lot else we could do, except make beds. I think humanism is part of the (M)odernist project... Incidentally I'm not saying that relationships aren't fundamental.

Sandy: Sometimes, I wish you wouldn't say anything.

Thesis for this chapter

- ❑ Postmodernist criticism emphasises that humanism, holism and positivism like any other philosophy rely upon metaphysical foundations that are open to argument. For example, humanism and freewill do not go hand in hand when nursing mentally ill young people and children
- ❑ Humanism and positivism utilise similar frameworks of language to categorise illness and approach. They can be clearly located within the wider context of Western metaphysics
- ❑ In the (M)odern sense, nursing specialities makes themselves unique by the materials they use, such as children and young people.

Background and aims

This chapter is concerned with humanism as a dominant philosophy/ideology and the process of caring as its perceived technology in practice. The first thing we debate is the notion that the process of caring (as delivered via humanistic practice within child and adolescent mental health) provides, in part, a unique role for nursing. The second points up the way psychiatry has taken over the concept of child-centred humanistic practice and yet hides and prioritises the conflicts inherent by such a synthesis of the two. Therefore, this chapter is concerned with two related issues. First, the nature of caring and humanism as a therapeutic framework for nursing and, second, the idea that such a framework is good enough to justify what it is we actually do as nurses (in an age of quantifiable care outcomes). Social agreement, autonomy, and freewill are concepts that form the core of humanistic philosophy and child-centred care, yet it is argued that these concepts are frequently misused and twisted to fit the actual facts. Humanistic child-centred care may be the dominant approach to child care and one that is largely beneficial, but that does not excuse us from the task of subjecting it to criticism. This chapter aims to:

1. Provide a working definition of humanism and an analysis of the concept of caring; and

2. Argue that humanism has served to lock nursing into an unsatisfactory status quo within child care.

Introduction: Humanism and nursing

What is humanism? In short, it is a collection of specific beliefs, doctrines about being human and, at its most intolerant, an ideology that is hypercritical of all that falls outside its own definition. As noted by Kolenda (1995: 340), humanism is 'a general perspective from which the world is viewed'; a perspective that is radically different from two other dominant beliefs about mankind—the supernatural and the biological. First, the supernatural, or divine order that assumes man was created by a divine being and has a determined position in a natural hierarchy; or second, the purely scientific, biological animal of a higher intelligence. Humanism distinguishes itself from these two by viewing mankind as possessing special and unique qualities that are not necessarily determined. Therefore, as noted by Kolenda (1995), it occupies a middle position between, on the one hand a divine and non-scientific order of the world, and a largely determined biological evolved order on the other.

Humanism as a doctrine is not new. It can be found in the writings of Plato and Aristotle and, in turn, was rediscovered through classical language and literature in the Renaissance. The term 'humanism' is younger and 'came into general use only in the nineteenth century, but was applied to intellectual and cultural developments in previous eras' (Kolenda, 1995). Traditionally, the philosophical basis for nursing and child development has been based upon a Judeo-Christian theology of, what Brykczynska (1995: 122) has called, 'professional idealism'. The move away from a starched uniform and supernatural emphasis towards humanism during the 1960s represented a radical shift in the direction of something that was considered modern and theoretically more stable. However, as also noted by Brykczynska (1995: 123), nurse theorists at the time provided theory that was 'haphazardly contradictory'. In an article written in a US nursing journal, attempting to explain humanism to nurses, Joseph (1985) states that the 'central tenets of humanism are not engraved in stone… the issues or tenants are evolving' (Brykczynska, 1995: 123). In contrast to this belief, Blackham (1963: 10) had already identified a number of essential concepts of humanism and he lists four that can be considered active ingredients of humanist philosophy:

1. Man is not naturally depraved;

2. The end of life is life itself, the good life on earth instead of the beatific life after death;
3. Man is capable, guided solely by the light of reason and experience, of perfecting the good life on earth; and
4. The first essential condition of the good life on earth is the freeing of men's minds from the bonds of ignorance and superstition, and of their bodies from the arbitrary oppression of the constituted social authorities.

These four guiding principles are those evident in much of the psychotherapy literature of the client-centred type. As such, they rely on two fundamental assumptions. First, patients' rights to informed consent and, secondly, consensus about the aims of the therapy.

In the past, the medical priority of seeking explanation for diseases and the nursing task of doing what doctor instructs, both tended to make patient consent and consensual therapy seem like pipe-dreams. More recently, however, there has been a rise in civil rights campaigns, the acceptance of the assumption that change must come from within, the belief in free information, advocacy, and self-care models of nursing. Such models include Paterson and Zderad's (1988) theory of nursing related to humanistic and existential concepts, which emphasises the need to understand the meaning of the patients' world and his/her relationship to society. This aim to demonstrate understanding is evident in Appleton (1993) and many other nursing models: they express humanistic client-centred care as the art of nursing, the 'doing' or creating of a therapeutic self. This created, or cloned 'therapeutic self' is, incidentally, a good example of three postmodern notions: the **reproduced** (or mass produced) commodity for use in nursing of **representation**, here of expertness, of professionalism, and also of **legitimisation**, in that, the therapeutic self appears to justify even our questionable practices in therapy.

Regarding society and the social agreement, it seems that there is little agreement about the social and moral functioning of what it is to be human. What is evident is that humanism holds that human beings become humanised via society; that is, they are socialised into the rules, rituals and customs of specific cultures. This constructionist view argues that, as humans, we are all obliged to conform to these certain rules in a kind of social contract. Society tends to ascribe the term 'mental illness' when there is a breakdown in 'normal' or acceptable human actions. Contact with psychiatry follows and society classifies or labels its deviant members via the expert gate keeper. As noted by Thompson and Mathias

(1994: 9), such an explanation has become open to abuse by lay persons and professionals as, 'much distress can be caused to families when it is suggested that a person's mental state is simply a way in which society classifies or labels its deviant members'. Thus highlighting the fact that postmodernist thought regarding psychiatric discourse and questioning the actual existence of mental illness may appear 'to be acceptable to an extent in academic terms, and having a value in explaining some of the experiences of a person with problems of illness and ill health, [but] the insensitive and inappropriate application of labelling theory may be of no consolation to those who see before them a loved family member disintegrating'. It is suggested by the authors that a sense of proportion is needed; the existence of postmodernist critique does not help these family members, neither does it obliterate the fact that labels and constructions of mental health are a reality. Many of the social institutions (such as the family) formed to protect children maybe disappearing (Plotz, 1988). It is, therefore, argued that a postmodernist critique offers alternative ways of thinking rather than solutions. The fact that all humans have feelings, emotions and experiences of differing intensity does not mean they are ill or experiencing the wrong things. This is a man-made construction. Perhaps the real question is one of individuality: that is, of how society contends with the labelled individual and how humanistic doctrine helps man to aid fellow man.

However, humanism has to accept that, as a set of specific beliefs regarding the individual, it does not rest comfortably with the notion of grand narratives regarding socialisation. It contends that the democratic social order is independent of ultimate and contentious beliefs (Blackham, 1963: 16). Co-operation on the grand or macro social scale creates that practicability for all that is the concrete content of freedom, a freedom that differs for mentally ill children and young people. Within humanist ethics, there is no far-off end of all action, only patterns of good living, or the attempt to attain virtue as one's own excellence. Hence the belief in achieving 'self actualisation' (Maslow, 1970) and one's 'full potential'. But, as noted by Blackham (1963: 19), the most material part of virtue is public spirit or a regard to the community. Therefore, although hedonism or the pleasure principle has been important in humanist ethics, it is stressed mainly because of the evil consequences of neglecting it. For nursing, humanism has become synonymous with patient interaction and guiding theoretical models. These include Peplau (1952/1988), Orem (1991) and Carl Rogers'

(1951) client-centred counselling. It emphasises a partnership and the need for patients to be self reliant. Hopton (1993) takes a more critical view by noting that humanistic psychology is often used to soften the impact of medicalisation on service users, especially children.

Overall, humanist philosophy provides us, as nurses working with mentally ill children and young people, with an approach that is seen to be pretty satisfactory. It encourages in us a belief that all children are individuals and worthy of respect regardless of gender, age, race, and background. It instils in us a belief that things can get better and that our patients can make self-determined choices that will affect care outcomes. It promotes beliefs that humans naturally cooperate in a form of social contract, irrespective of power or hierarchical issues. As an approach, it allows for a demonstration of respect, warmth, and acceptance (as we are taught in the schools of nursing). It is a very congenial approach because it emphasises virtue and tolerance. All children are good and can get better given the right nurture and guidance. This is simplistic humanist thought. However, the reverse of the coin leads us to the constructionist position that there can only be limited self-determinism in a society and social reality, which are governed by large structures and powerful discourses. For example, how self-determined can a young person be when he/she is labelled mentally ill? As an approach, humanism fits very well within the realms of the more scientific boundaries of holism, as discussed in the previous chapter. Holism, in the nursing sense, promotes the theory and practice of treating the child as a whole person rather than just as parts. It is assumed to be strongly anti-reductionist, but is, in fact, on the reductionist scale unless viewed as specifically **person** holist. To treat a child holistically is assumed to be good humanist practice. It demonstrates our virtue and makes allowances for children's behaviour because we are sensitive to wider issues. Therefore, (as shown in the figure below) humanism seems to be the perfect supporting act, both for holism and for the knowledge base of nursing discussed in the previous chapter. But the very success of humanism in this highly technocratic age arouses postmodern suspicion— the apparent difficulty of finding criticisms of humanism leads us to think that it is not addressed to real issues; (as noted by Pursey), its naive optimism makes the authors of the book charge humanism with being a surface philosophy—not least because it has little to say to nurses who feel subordinated to a wholly medicalised psychiatry, or who are sensitive to the concealed (but undeniable) power imbalance between nurse and young person. In short, it is criticised for irrationally proposing that its core tenets of freewill, autonomy, social agreement, and ethics can be shaped and moulded into something that resembles child-centred care. As noted by Blackham (1963a: 103), 'the most drastic objection to humanism is that it is too bad to be true'.

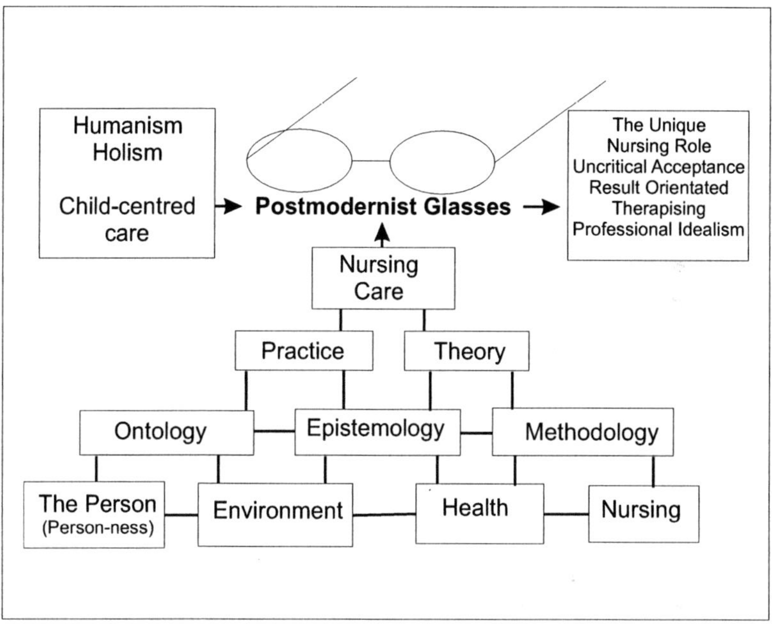

Figure 3.1: The building blocks of nursing theory.

Humanism and the concept of caring

When we look backwards in order to move forwards, we are only re-thinking the assumptions held to be fact by most nurses. It is a commonly held belief that humanism is a modern philosophy for nursing and it is one that has come to dominate the development of nurse-patient interpersonal models of care. It is taken for granted that, at present, it is the best philosophy for nursing young people and one that takes into account many theoretical issues. These include the re-humanising of the medical process, the advocacy of individualism—with its phenomenological aspirations, including personal agency and the promotion of professional value judgements. In order to show that humanism has, in fact, been accepted by nurses unconditionally, it is necessary to critically analyse the language, concepts, and value judgements that have made it successful, or at least so plausible. As a philosophy that seems to be human focussed and, therefore, child focussed, its alliance to the phenomenological spheres of thought places it, at first glance, in opposition to structural theories of determinism and free will. It is on this issue of freewill that we will now focus and follow it by a critique of humanism's other core concepts of social agreement and of its metaphysics. Each in turn will be critically analysed. This type of devil's advocacy has the aim of illuminating issues worthy of further discussion throughout this book. It is emphasised that, as with most postmodernist experimental criticism, no solutions or opposites will be put forward. Whereas the (M)odern aimed to provide certainty and progress, the postmodern appears to create uncertainty in what we believe to be true.

Freewill and autonomy

For the purpose of this discussion, the term 'freewill' relates to the internal ability of a child or young person to make decisions (rather than the philosophical debate arising from cause and effect generally). Autonomy refers to that choice bestowed upon the child by another. We mean that freedom to choose that others (nurses, here) assumed the young person does have, must have—which sometimes they **insist** the young person has and **must exercise**. As previously noted by Blackham (1963), a founding principle of humanism is its insistence that all men are free to make the good life for themselves, based upon their capabilities of reason. A reason that is founded in the belief that the universe is crossed by a web of correspondences that tie man's nature and the fate of individual men and women to the natural world (Smith, 1997: 49). Therefore, the ability to make 'the good life' depends upon what it is to be natural and what it is to be moral, or social. As Isidore of Seville observed in the seventh century, 'The human race is ruled in two ways, by nature and by custom' (Smith, 1997: 86). For nursing practice, this poses the question, How effective can a therapeutic relationship with a young person be, if the child or young person has no real personal autonomy or free will? There may be no definite answer to this question, but it is proposed by the authors that nurses too often take it for granted that they must allow the young person autonomy—at least in principle. However, the gap between our principles as nurses and what we have to do in practice reminds us that a shared or rationed autonomy is at best an incoherent idea; at worst, it may be a form of oppression. In any case, it disguises itself as a notion of self-care and equal partnership. It is also important to note how different a child's needs are from those of an older adolescent: reality ('my own truth about reality') is differently perceived by each and, therefore, different for each. The question then, may be not one of asking how to provide the child with more autonomy, but rather one that examines the wider structures which constrain us all. As noted by Lather (1990: 101), 'A post-humanist theory of the subject [in this postmodern period] combines Derrida's critique of the metaphysics of presence with a post-Althusserean focus on human agency'. As such, this translates into a search for subjectivity within the written word (e.g. textbooks, articles, and the like) about choice and freewill for young people in hospital as a cultural product. In this case, these cultural products usually relate to the obvious age and legal obligations, the professional and cultural obligations that are seen to protect both the young person and the nurse. These are nursing objectives, which are seen as being relevant to the mainstream structures needed for health, recovery and, what Lather (1990: 101) describes as, a 'site for potential change'. This echoes Maslow's (1970) call for growth towards self-actualisation. Also, perhaps the child's autonomy is not necessary for a trusting relation to be founded between a dependent child and an all powerful nurse. Is the ability to trust a consequence of being able to make executive decisions? The answer is, obviously, no. Perhaps the wrong questions are being asked—a criticism made of other methods of analysis—and they have naturally pointed us toward the view that autonomy is beneficial to a young person's care outcomes. Are nurses being asked to make ethical decisions regarding what is a reasonable quality or quantity of autonomy, so that learning by the client can take place, so that 'full potential' can be realised? If this is the case, child-centred care is not grounded in humanism regarding the issue of freewill. Not all children and young people in nurses' care will want autonomy or will be able to bear it.

As a core objective, the concept of autonomy and the acceptance of personal responsibility is seen as being the overriding aim of most nursing interventions. The issue of decentering the subject, which is a central theme in postmodern thought, will be discussed in greater detail in *Section III*, but for now, it is important to note that, in practice, nurses hardly ever hand over significant responsibility to their young patients. Young people and children (unlike older adult patients) have very little if any choice about treatment. Thus, they have very little autonomy to make choices or engage in the practice of responsibility. This may appear to be an obvious and unavoidable consequence of age, but it is one that is inseparable in child and adolescent mental health nursing. It is also one that, as yet, is often tackled in practice utilising adult nursing frameworks.

We need to remember that the speciality needs to define itself by the nature of its being. By that we mean that the issues of autonomy, self-care, or health promotion, and many others, might just be practical myths. It emphasises that the deciding upon central nursing aims are not necessarily child-centred, but nurse led and perhaps this is not a bad thing. Such is the importance of the determinist-free will debate that it is worthy of discussion regarding the nature of caring in child and adolescent mental health nursing. The issue of autonomy, as a universal commodity, is promoted in the modernist Utopia as an expected and guaranteed right of all. These rules do not necessarily apply to children and young people, and form part of a wider issue of the social agreement among the millions of individuals in the world.

Social agreement

The social agreement, in humanist terms, is an important concept that attempts to provide answers to questions about how humans should relate to one another. It is a code of moral practice urging men and women to attempt to live the good life and promote the full potential of self and their fellow man. The social agreement for nursing, as an ethical principle, is perceived by the majority of the public as being something about caring. Caring, in turn, is perceived as being something essential to nursing, done by nurses. It is that which distinguishes nursing from other health professions. It is a process and involves a moral stance. Primarily, it requires the nurse to be competent and safe. It is the ethical foundation for nursing and, according to Watson (1988: 29), it is the moral ideal of nursing whereby the outcome is the protection, enhancement, and preservation of human dignity. There are a number of authors who recognise two dimensions of caring. One is instrumental and the other is affective, i.e. either directed to achieving a practical result (biological comfort) or a change in mental state (mental comfort). However, caring also has a limiting effect in nursing, as noted by Hall (1990), who said that nursing care described technical and hotel service activities carried out by nurses. This argument reminds us that many nurses sometimes feel they are a baby-sitting service or just substitute parents, as they attempt to provide a professional standard of care for their young patients. This notion is also very peculiar to child and adolescent nursing and one that determines the approach of much nursing care. Existing theories of caring are not empirically adequate for generating the hypotheses about staff behaviours that are essential for good care. Therefore, caring as a concept is usually subordinated to the process of interaction and actual contact with young people. It is synonymous with the approaches typified by phrases, such as, 'If I didn't care, I wouldn't enforce the unit rules' approach, or 'I care enough to make time to see you'. As such, caring is a fundamental component of holistic nursing practice. Child-centred caring is tangled up in a social agreement among nurses, stating that nursing is about caring if nothing else. Nurses have a duty to be caring.

Continuing with this theme of duty to care, Kitson (1993) noted there are three ways of conceptualising caring. These are:

1. Caring as a duty;
2. Caring as therapy; and
3. Caring as an ethical position.

The notion of caring is seen as a central issue to the unique contribution of nursing, because it provides the basis for 'the art of nursing', that is what we do in practice. The work of Appleton (1993) highlights five distinct meta-themes that express the art of nursing. The issue of caring is a core facet to all five, as a distinct and unique nursing role. Her phenomenological and, therefore, constructivist approach, as she notes, is 'particularly suited for discovering the art of nursing', because it 'reveals the art of nursing from the lived experience of the patient and the nurse'. Such experience takes into account the fact that a relationship (between two people) can be experienced as itself existing, as being and changing, as being a thing distinguishable from the people involved. The use of the therapeutic self is widely assumed to be central to the nurse-patient interface in mental health nursing, hence the importance given to the humanistic perspective. As such, the knowledge base of nursing as an art borrows heavily from humanist as well as holist philosophy. A discussion regarding the nature of caring and humanist philosophy has the purpose of exploring the epistemology of nursing and the nature of determinism in it, and will prove useful when discussing the expansion of the child and adolescent nursing knowledge base in the following chapters.

The framework for understanding many of the issues related to choice and free will in the child-nurse caring relationship capitalises on the contact and communication process. The art of nursing differs between adult and child nursing as just discussed, but also because it focusses on the lived experience of each individual's own sense of being (ontology). It is this focus that, in the realist sense, reformulates our conception of knowledge and, therefore, free will by moving the emphasis back from what it is to know, to focus on what it is to be. Realist approaches, according to Wainwright (1997), have an ontology, stating that the structures creating the world cannot be directly observed; the only real truths are those experienced through being. It is with this sense of being that the art of nursing has its foundations. The following are the five meta-themes of the art of nursing offered by Appleton (1993):

1. The way of being there in caring;
2. The way of being within understanding caring;
3. The way of creating opportunities for fullness of being through caring;
4. A transcendent togetherness; and
5. The context of caring.

It is with the first that we now continue our analysis.

Just being there in caring—the unique nursing role

Being there in caring is the single most important aspect of the art of nursing recognised by nurses and young people. By being there in the actual and metaphysical sense, the nurse is demonstrating both humanist and existential qualities, such as accepting the whole child who has fears and a connected life beyond the need for care. The child is unique, and the being there in terms of relationship building is different on each occasion for child and nurse; this emphasises the child-centeredness within the personal connectedness of the process. The idea of just being there within the notion of the art of nursing may seem simple and obvious, but it is unique to the role of the nurse and is not so clearly seen in the work of other MDT professionals. When a child is upset in Tier 4, the nurse is often the comforter. In other tiers, it is the nurse who attempts to initiate and establish a relationship in order that containment can be established for healing and caring. When a young person is scared and fears a lack of control, it is usually the nurse who is there embodying the caring process. There is nothing scientific or medical about hugging a distraught, angry child. In this sense, humanism is a position and not a philosophy; it is not in need of metaphysics because it cannot take sides on the big metaphysical issues of design or purpose in the Universe. It holds that caring is a way of being, a way to demonstrate the good life, a way to view the individual who is trying to make sense of his/her own existence in a confusing reality.

This leads to an idea of connectedness, a 'way of being within understanding caring'. In a similar way to Peplau's (1952/1988) working phase, the way of understanding care is the art of sharing the development of the nurse-child relationship. It is well recognised by mainstream nursing theory that building trust enables relationships to develop and the nurse to discover uniqueness in the patient in ways that are not necessarily scientifically predictable. Nursing, within the realms of child and adolescent mental health, is unique because it explores the nature of care, and what it means to the child, with the aim of building a relationship, so that care can be thought through and given attentively to the child. This investment of personal involvement is also uniquely found in nursing, and emphasises the importance of time spent with young people. As noted by Appleton (1993), 'patients found that nurses create nursing by taking time to care and by giving their very best'. Nurses invest themselves. They don't prescribe medication or diagnose as a central part of their role. In general, nurses don't have special set-aside times to be with and formally 'help' a child; the longer periods of contact give them the flexibility to match interventions to occasions. They don't step into the child's life for an hour a week in an attempt to 'fix' the problem; rather they are there for and with the child in need.

The specific interventions that are built into most residential health care units (Tier 4) and community settings (Tiers 3 and 2) involve the skills of nurses who 'create opportunities for the fullness of being' through the process of caring. The truism that children and young people should have a degree of responsibility for growth acknowledges their individuality, life experiences, and fears for the future. The nurse is involved in finding ways for them to achieve, or even discover their aims, and assist them to find their unique way out of their particular situation. This involves helping them make responsible decisions and guiding self-expression. The difficulty of making the safe passage lies within the humanistic framework, that is, promoting growth towards full potential. The safe passage through developmental and transition periods emphasises the need for nurses to create new opportunities to advance nursing practice; clearly, young people experiencing mental illness will find development especially hard to negotiate.

'A transcendent togetherness' portrays the liberating process of an emancipatory relationship that develops in the art of nursing. The issue of liberation is seen as something intrinsically linked to nursing in the eyes of many young people. It concerns the personal transformations of both nurse and child as the caring process proceeds. The transformation is very evident in the community setting, where a young person views his/her time and contact with the nurse as being potent and his/her own. Nursing is the primary source of care, and care consists in valuing. It may be argued that the notion of nursing's 'art' has just shifted the emphasis of care delivery, repackaged it, and called it something new. Other critics emphasise the limitations of humanist philosophy, first, as a foundation to provide a complete and concise model of care and, second, to do what it aims, that is, value children as individuals and provide a child-centred approach. The art of nursing is a knowledge base that is uniquely nursing. It sits comfortably within the meta-paradigm of nursing and offers a platform from which practice can be advanced. But within this notion of a unique role for nurses, there are further criticisms that can be raised, including the issue of humanist commitment.

Humanist commitment

As noted by Blackham (1963: 26), humanist commitment is about answering the question, 'What do you do ?' Is it true to say that to practice in a humanist, child-centred way is to be more than ordinarily honest-minded, accepting, tolerant? We all practice our counselling skills, we use reflective practice and video work to improve our interpersonal skills, so that Carl Rogers himself would applaud us. We, as nurses, have demonstrated an unconditional acceptance of child-centred care. We assume that it is the best possible position from which to utilise our therapeutic selves. The technology, which is evident in other spheres of nursing, such as defibs, dialysis machines, and operating theatres, is not applicable to the speciality of child and adolescent mental health nursing. We are not really mistaken in not presenting any tools of a trade in order to justify our unique roles. All we have, and have always had, is ourselves. We attempt to specialise the process of listening and giving advice, then label these new phenomena as counselling and psychotherapy. We call listening, active listening and talking, paraphrasing. We use protocols and models that share common research and historical origins based in the humanities—the humanist tradition—to hide this very plain and unadorned fact: that all we have as nurses caring for ill children is ourselves to offer. As a community, we don't hum and buzz like a technologically advanced machine, and this has always given us cause for concern.

The authors argue that we are committed to the humanistic child-centred care process not solely because it is beneficial to the young person, but because we have to justify our role somehow. It is the rational rather than the irrational approach that is a product of culture and (in our era) (M)odernity. In a world where more means best and order means success, it seems obvious and rational for us, as nurses, to rely upon humanist approaches that are acceptable to the majority because of their soft interface (that is, their interpersonal friendliness). In nursing, and especially the nursing of young people and children, nurses can be considered a culturally-produced product, which is seen above all else as caring; the cultural production of perceived caring professionals is seen as a good thing. It is ethically unsound to swear at or tell a child that you don't like them; this is not a good thing; it does not harbour the duty-bound ethics of humanist goodness, ethics that make us feel safe and, perhaps, even stupid when, according to our supervisors, we can't seem to get the advanced empathy right. As a historical artefact, such considerations of professional conduct can be seen to transcend the way we conceptualise reason as always existing in the humanist sense in the individual. This is (M)odernity in question, because humanistic principles, such as good manners, professional conduct, and the care of children as they grow and develop, is a recent phenomenon. And the psychotherapeutic assumption that the mind is something individual and able to be exercised via humanistic counselling is also recent. As noted by Parker *et al* (1995: 13), the fascination in Western culture with the idea that there is an integrated self-conscious core to the human being, and that it must be possible to discover this 'presence' lying in every person, reiterates the modernist wish to critique adequately the concepts and language used to underpin the metaphysical assumptions we take for granted.

We are committed to child-centred caring because it allows us to be self-sufficient, separate, and distinct. It is the humanising of the science of nursing and *vis versa.* As proclaimed specialists of the interpersonal domain, we profess to cure those presences inside and bring them out. For modernity also brings with it the classification of experiences, which child-centred care promotes. As noted by Parker *et al* (1995: 13), the common core of both medical and psychoanalytical variants of psychiatric practice is that the abnormal is experienced as something internal to the person. Foucault (1971) calls to our attention the notion of the confession. Counselling reduces all experiences to a moral judgement. Humanism has the aim of respecting all men and assuming we all have the intention to aspire to goodness. The fact we are all human also means we make value judgements about the behaviours of other fellow men. Child psychiatry has the role of policing such judgements, which are very often assumed to be produced from family dynamics and environmental factors. As noted by Parker *et al* (1995: 18) 'psychoanalytic theory offers an interesting and attractive constructionist view of the self; it seduces many radicals in mental health work into accepting, at the same time, reactionary therapeutic practices carried out in its name'.

Demand-centred care

The modernist preoccupation with commodity and surplus supply allows us to recognise that humanist child-centred practice is in demand. As an alternative to other 'psychiatric therapies', which often include the use of medication and ECT, it is viewed as a better option, one that can be added onto by combining various forms of therapy. It is, therefore, multi purposeful and able to meet the needs of many regardless of each one's individuality. It is the softer option, which should be available to all, and is because of the limited rivals. As nurse therapists, we tempt the counselled into needing the recognition of others to help suppress any doubts they may have about their own independent existence. Perhaps the presenting problems don't exist, but we try to locate them or (as noted by Thomas Szasz, 1961) pretend they exist. Therefore, it is quite possible that child-centred care manifests itself by its own condition and relation to (M)odernism and the demand culture we all live in. When a parent tells a psychiatrist anxiously that she has heard that there are all sorts of therapies available and surely one of them would help her little girl, the easy option is to surmise or create a problem and therapise it. Even if there is an obvious problem, such as school refusal or bed wetting, it is still an option to therapise it. Assessment and therapising go hand in hand, because, as already noted, these are all the tools we have, and it is these tools that give mental health nursing the tools that validate the remit of mental health nursing. The mystifying language of these supposed therapies titillates parents into believing they are capable of rescuing their depressed young sons and daughters. The unrealistic expectations asked of humanistic child-centred counselling often reiterates its own limitations in an age in which everything seems so certain. If nothing else, a study of the postmodern highlights that nothing is certain and that the language we use structures the way we think.

Power

The unequal power relationship within psychotherapeutic relationships has been noted by Masson (1990), in particular, the way the practice of psychotherapy manipulates and controls the interaction process. Within the realms of child and adolescent mental health care, the nurse as the responsible adult has the fact of power to overcome in an attempt to provide humanistic child-centred care. Regardless of where (in which tier service) the therapeutic relationship is processed, the nurse will always be viewed as the authority figure, the superior, the helper, and so on. While this power imbalance is usually acknowledged and accounted for, it emphasises some of the difficulties just explored and highlighted. Namely, that there is no such thing as child-led care, only psychiatric-led care. On a more optimistic note, it should be said that caring can be thought of as something distinct from treating, although related to it. And this, perhaps, lies at the heart of what we intend when we try to provide quality nursing care. Nurses treat because of the nature of their role in tier service provision. We are paid to treat and we can be paid to care. However, this last clause is still an aspiration.

Fading remarks

This chapter has scratched the surface of two major concerns for nursing relating to the consequences of child-centred care and humanism. Humanism's growth within psychiatry has offered a model based upon the practical principles of client-centred psychotherapies. The philosophy of humanism is thought to guide and determine action. This action aims to create an equalness between the nurse and child within a unique relationship. This notion that all humans are unique and have the ability to make decisions is doubly troublesome for nurses working with young people. First, the notion of uniqueness (see United Kingdom Central Council for Nursing, Midwifery, and Health

Visiting, 1992) is not achievable. The possibility that young people can be treated as unique is a debate that alone could take a whole book. The wish to treat patients as unique has dominated nursing literature (Johnson and Smith, 1994: 25), but is also what Brykczynska (1995: 122) has called 'professional idealism'. The move away from the starched uniform and supernatural emphasis of God-li-ness ushered in a belief in humanism, a fitting philosophy for an age dominated by man as opposed to nature. Such a shift shows us that culture has a relationship with nursing that is sometimes not so obvious to detect.

Section II: The modernist project

Aims for this section

(1) To highlight the way modern nursing has adopted a scientific and manufacturing agenda from other disciplines in order to provide itself with professional boundaries, thus protecting its limited power and the progress assimilated with having more;

(2) To show how nursing has adopted a multi paradigmatic theory to underwrite its limited professional power, and how this has provided a distinct nursing ideology; and

(3) From a culture of progress comes the best a culture can offer : Advanced nursing practice—a symbol of all that is modern.

Chapter 4
Professionalising the process—processing the profession

"The importance of having reliable assessment instruments and diagnosis has long been acknowledged in the medical treatment of children"

(Rey *et al*, 1989)

Dialogue

Dean: But what if things were different...Say there wasn't such thing as specialism or a thing...

Sandy: Uhm...

Dean: I mean that the nursing process belongs to the realms of logic, it's modern. It tries to objectify everything we do...at the same time it's all we've got.

Sandy: So?

Dean: Well...the processing of nursing duties is an attempt to modernise and professionalise that which we do. They seem to go hand in hand.

Sandy: What are you saying? Don't you think science in nursing is a good thing?

Dean: I think that science is often thought of as the producer of progress. In much the same way, nursing generally has attempted to legitimise its role through a process, one that is advertised as being scientifically objective.

Sandy: So what?

Dean: Well, so nothing, it's just an interesting phenomenon isn't it. One that illuminates the power we think things like the nursing process have in defining how we care for young people.

Thesis for this chapter

- ❑ (M)odernity in nursing is essentially about advancement and a quest for professional autonomy. A legitimisation of 'Nursing-as-a- Profession'
- ❑ Child and adolescent mental health nursing has boundaries that always take into account the nature of the unique nature of our materials, e.g. age and development issues. However, child and adolescent mental health nursing relies totally upon adult models of psychiatry as a way of ordering practice
- ❑ Diagnosis and classifications comprise a language that is socially constructed and bears no resemblance to reality. They are more likely to be concerned with power issues than with caring.

Background and aims

This chapter aims to explore some of the broader issues related to nursing 'professionalism', issues that have a direct consequence upon child and adolescent mental health nursing. In many ways, it mirrors some of the issues discussed throughout this section, because it is ultimately assumed that, in order to develop child and adolescent mental health nursing, the speciality has to have expanded practice, be it at a grass roots level or politically. This chapter has three aims:

1. To discuss the perceived boundaries of nursing as they are at present;
2. To explore the rise of new nursing—a new modernism; and
3. To begin to identify the boundaries of the specialism.

Introduction: The promotion of specialism

Boundaries signify the extent to which a group of professionals consider their remit begins and ceases. These boundaries are related to actual clinical practice, academia, management, and research. Nurses seem to be unable to agree upon the extent to which nursing has a growing, yet distinct epistemology, ontology, and methodology. Also, our trade cannot agree on the direction in which any theoretical and practice expansion should progress, thus highlighting the incompatibility between nurses who believe specialism and fragmentation to be the only way forward, and those who argue for a unified generalism or foundationalism, in order to justify a status of professionalism. The issue of a unified paradigm of nursing academia and research is ambiguous, as already discussed (see *Chapter 2*), but, according to Ellis and Hartley (1992), nurse theorists and nurse researchers are of the opinion that the profession of nursing has its own body of knowledge. Our question is, Has child and adolescent mental health? And our answer is, No. Although we assume it ought to have, we must acknowledge that practice relevant in adult settings is usually utilised in child and adolescent nursing. The use of the therapeutic self, seclusion, ward rounds, and environment (milieu therapy-issues of containment/community living/respect for self and others) are as universal to this specialised care setting as any other. Family therapy is one of the few interventions (apart from the increased attempts to provide a homely environment and less dependency upon medication) that child and adolescent services seem to claim for their own. This, then, is an argument that promotes the specialisation of distinct nursing areas in order to provide more focussed theory-based practice. As such, demonstrating a thorough knowledge of the science and art of nursing, as well as the ability to recognise phenomena and the ability to create new concepts. Within this belief in specialisation, the goal of nursing can still be seen as searching for information about health, the individual, the environment and well being of the total person (child), coupled with the promotion of the health of the community. However, it is apparent that nursing, in its strive for modernisation, would view postmodern knowledge as a chaotic notion that, ultimately, has the one objective of distracting its march towards legitimisation and modernist respectability in the eyes of its multi-disciplinary colleagues. As such, postmodern thought can be seen as a radical threat, a threat that undermines the possibility of nursing being a naturally occurring phenomena—a phenomena that is in control of its still undecided small portion of reality with, according to Kvale (1990: 2), 'notions of language as actually constituting the structures of a perspectival social reality'. Such a perspectival reality encompasses the idea of specialism in its localised sense, because 'the dichotomy of universal social laws and the individual self is replaced by the interaction of local networks' (Kvale, 1990: 3). Therefore, the specialism of child and adolescent mental health nursing, apart from being considered an efficient unit of production in terms of a modernist health trade framework, can also be heralded as a postmodern formulation, that is, it has the potential, like other specialisms, to be sidetracked from the path of enlightened reason in the search for universal truths, and might concern itself with the concepts of power and knowledge in terms of mental health and nursing young people. With this in mind, it is necessary to explore the current position in which all the tiers of child and adolescent mental health nurses currently find themselves.

Pluralism in nursing

There is a difference in the goals of the nurses, managers, statuary boards, and academics. One of the oldest and most talked about differences is the rift between the so called 'theory-practice gap'. This is a byproduct of the modernist need to justify, rationalise, and account theoretically for all human behaviour. Although not altogether healthy, it motivates the debate and articulates the differences between professional wants and needs within a professional whole. The profession of nursing continues to be dominated by generalist practitioners, if only because of their numbers. Among the generalists is a large cohort who maintain that their occupation is a practical one. The idea of specialism co-habits uncomfortably with the widespread expectation that all nurses will have a broadly similar skill mix applicable to most areas of nursing. Within this belief, there is the notion that nurses who have spent many years practising within a particular setting (for example, child and adolescent mental health) will exhibit advanced skills based upon experience and exposure to many emotionally demanding situations. Such an assumption has to bear in mind the need for theoretical reflection. The growth in recent years of the specialist camp is coupled with demands for increased professional accountability and authority, and a belief that nursing can develop a 'science of caring'. The demands are made in the belief that all must aim at a goal of securing an objective and global system of knowledge that represents reality; that will be the legitimation—as sought by all other professional groups—that will secure professionalism for nursing as a whole. Science is seen as this standard of progress and measured against the backdrop of technological advances. This has recently come to be known as 'new nursing'. Professional bodies, such as the RCN, support the specialists, but are thwarted by the ideologies of managers and generalists who make up most of their membership. In particular, ideologies that view anything non-(M)odern as ineffectual romanticism, themselves hinder the achievement of practical objectives.

In child and adolescent mental health, the specialisation of this client group has evolved due to the push of psychiatry. That push has secured its ideological domination and all-powerful medicalising over the care provision provided to this group. This reminds us of Habermas's (1971) insight that there is ideology present in all spheres of human culture. This is especially true if such ideology is necessary for a dominant group to obtain power and remain secure in expressing it. On the other hand, nursing as an official role, as noted by Heideman and Crabbe (1991), was a 'mixture of modified 'mother's role' activities, discipline of patients and custodial companionship care'. That mother role is evidently shaped by Peplau's (1989) theories of the therapeutic use of self. Here we have another example of child and adolescent nursing being built upon adult mental health frameworks. As if still tied to the apron strings, Fagin (1972) described the role of child psychiatric nurses as intervening to:

1. Assist children with new learning;
2. Assist children and their families with relearning roles, relationships and expectations; and
3. Assist in restoring deprived aspects of living (cited in Heideman and Crabbe, 1991: 5).

As such, the assumption that nurses practising within this speciality are child-centred is the driving force behind specialisation (as we have already shown). Coupled with the many reports of specific needs for this client group, nursing has taken time to catch up with the political momentum that heralded the new age of specialism. It was during the 1970s that specialism was acknowledged in both the USA and the UK. The association, Advocates for Child Psychiatric Nursing (1971) and the ANA Council on Psychiatric and Mental Health Nursing developed a speciality group on child and adolescent issues in the USA. In the UK, separate units in London, Birmingham and Manchester were formally opened to admissions.

It is easy to be seduced into the belief that child and adolescent mental health nursing is fully a specialism when compared to others, and there is no doubt that, as a result of the age of modernism and the relationship nursing has with psychiatry, the development of the specialism has succeeded in meeting some of the objectives it set out to do during the twentieth century. However, what if these objectives were not the right ones? What if other, alternative modes of production or definitions of what nursing ought to be were lost under the dominant discourses of psychiatry, and its promise to protect us all from the new leprosy of mental illness? Perhaps there will never be an answer to these questions, but it is safe to surmise that nursing, with its fragmented specialism, has had no choice but to adopt the modern model of development. It has been confined like nearly all others to take its place within the hierarchy of professions; a hierarchy that has placed, and will continue to place, emphasis upon progress and, therefore, stands fast upon logical and metaphysical foundations. Its quest for autonomy (even if displaced in localised specialities) leads to a failure to acknowledge new ways of conceptualising itself. Instead, the prospect of continued fragmentation and a determined belief in, and adoption of, psychiatric discourse ensures that it will remain secondary to psychiatry, less powerful, and with its boundaries of influence constrained by those of psychiatry. We will now look deeper into the issue of nursing's fragmentation.

Types of fragmentation

The issue of fragmentation involves the chance of increased power for select elites. Unfortunately, if nurses are divided into distinct specialisms, there is a tendency to over-emphasise differences between the different types of patients—or illness—they care for, to the exclusion of any overlap, similarity, or mere common humanity that patients have. One only has to look at the path of midwifery to find a living example. Nurses often talk about rehab, acute or elderly, as though each is a specialised entity. In this sense, each grouping seems to form a naturally occurring boundary related, first, to the type of client group and, second, to the nature of the nursing skills necessary. There is an associated status within these and this begins to reveal the underlying nursing ideology. For the newly qualified nurse, there is an expectation that acute nursing will benefit career pathways, whereas working with the elderly could limit choices (if stuck on a 'backwater' ward)—hence the rush to work in acute areas. For child and adolescent nursing, there is an ideology that assumes nurses within this specialism provide something, or have qualities that are uniquely useful to, or applied to, this client group. It is also assumed that these 'somethings' are determined by the nature of the clients. The point in question, however, is that such 'somethings' belong to all specialisms. As previously discussed, we know that caring is the unique quality of nursing that separates it from other professions. The question now is, What makes child and adolescent nursing a specialism? The answer is the nature of its client group and that alone. Consider Greenberg's (1980) assertion that modernism is somehow related to the materials that are used in its production; with this in mind, it would be naive to believe that any other unlearned quality separates a nurse practitioner in adolescent mental health from any other speciality. All the assumptions regarding the quality of the individual nurse have to be assessed against the back drop of a commitment to empirical, theoretical knowledge. One example is the need to utilise developmental theory to understand how a child thinks and behaves. Although knowing such information helps us, as nurses, legitimise our role, it is also fair to say that anyone with reasonable cognition who is capable of reading would be able to grasp such concepts. To rely on the assumption that this nursing specialism is anything more than learned skills is a falsehood. Even more, it is a myth that is perpetuated in order to maintain a degree of power and solidarity. By solidarity, the authors refer to the idea that child and adolescent nursing as a speciality is highly dependant upon theoretical paradigms of adult mental nursing, developmental theories, biological, and social sciences. We argue, therefore, that fragmentation is largely an illusion; after all, most mental health nurses share the same body of knowledge and understanding of it when they practice. As noted by Beck *et al* (1987), child mental health nurses 'also draw on theories, such as systems, symbolic interactions, communication, interpersonal, learning, psychoanalysis, stress, and crisis'.

The point in question is that, as a specialism, child and adolescent mental health nursing has to expand its own boundaries. If we believe (as most other text books on child and adolescent nursing will have it) that nursing is autonomous, then we are easily fooled. It is these same textbooks that promote a psychiatric model, full of medical diagnosis and discourse. Not only has nursing a responsibility to itself and to the young people, but also to society at large. This broad arena has to incorporate an ideology that promotes specialism as progress. Any suggested change or belief is legitimated by the motive of improved nursing care, of patient-centredness, and by less altruistic agendas. Nurse-speak currently propounds 'research awareness' and 'evidence based practice'. Parse (1981) also affirms nursing's responsibility to society. The responsibility to society is to guide the 'choosing of possibilities in the changing health process' implying that nurses should also be involved in political debate and policy making regarding health care provision. However, the major preoccupation of nursing continues to be its misguided attempt to achieve professionalisation.

The professionalisation of nursing

Sometimes nursing is referred to as a profession. This implies a certain level of expertise and education, which supports that expertise, and control over the application of that expertise in practice. Efforts to achieve this control have been referred to as the 'professional project' (Witz, 1991 ; MacDonald, 1995). There is a strong case for arguing that for nurses in the UK, the professional project has failed (Gavin, 1997). Yet the idea of professionalism remains an important part of the development of nursing in the late twentieth century. The landscape of nursing has been greatly altered in recent years by the 'market'. What nursing is and who defines the boundaries are recurring questions. Certain answers may have the ability to upset the specialism apple cart. The answers to these questions are tied up in nursing's relationship with society at large. It is socially constructed (Barker *et al*, 1995)—it is 'mediated' by the state (MacDonald, 1995: 134). Nurses who pursue the professional project are attempting to persuade the public and politicians that nurses should be given more power over their practice and to accept their ideological justifications for autonomy. If nursing is ever to achieve its professional project and emerge from subordination to others, and achieve an independent source of legitimacy (Rushing, 1993), then it must clarify its own ideology and persuade society of its value, and the worth of its values. These include a commitment to the role of science and to the concept of caring. Hamilton (1992: 32) defines professionalisation as '...the process by which an occupation develops the characteristics of a profession...'. Carter (1994) identifies nurses own resistance to change as a reason for their reluctance to move from traditional practices towards confrontation with male-dominated ideologies.

Professional identity

If we accept that the nursing care of children and adolescents did not just appear, then it belongs to a long history of human culture that includes developments in nursing generally, medicine, psychiatry, education, and social welfare. It would be wise, therefore, to assume it reflects trends and dominant discourses that carry traces of past discourses. According to Hector (1982), modern nursing began in the middle of the nineteenth century. However, as noted by other scholars (Lister, 1997; Sarup, 1988), modern times began earlier with the Enlightenment. This period, with its new liberalism, we can describe with historical perspective as modern. It sought to apply logic, reason, and science to all man's activities. Changes in society, especially the industrial revolution and its Marxist critique, reasoned that science had become applied to prejudice, nationalism, and power-seeking politics; politics that had their foundations firmly in the metaphysical beliefs and expectation of continual progress towards a better future. Nursing has always participated in this belief that science and medicine during the twentieth century can right all ills. In particular, mental health nursing is inseparable from psychiatry. The psychiatric discourse socialises participants into stereotypes, usually with doctors telling nurses what to do. Fundamental to the socialisation process, is the internalisation of values, norms, and ethical standards of the professional culture. Professionalism is seen as a framework used by professionals to place their work in a social role context. Perception of the professional self focusses on personal attributes that are considered to influence how the actual role-contents are performed. 'Nurse-speak' champions this self awareness (reflective practice-critical incident techniques, etc). Therefore, it is argued that consideration of legitimising strategies for child and adolescent nursing is pluralistic in nature and that its nursing ideology is concerned with economy, status and the power of specialism. This relates to the position children and young people occupy in society generally. However, a distinction should be drawn between the public view of cancer in childhood and mental health problems in childhood. One only has to take a look through a few inches of coverage in national newspapers to appreciate that they seem to be worlds apart—and wards apart too. It is obvious that mental health services are usually considered low priority when compared to other more pressing issues, such as chemotherapy for gravely ill children. Besides, the world as mediated by news editors, with headlines, such as, 'These children just needs to learn some manners'. But this leaves us with a serious dilemma, if the larger world outside child and adolescent services does not seem to care how political nursing should be?

New nursing—New professionalism: An ideological view into the future

Although child and adolescent nursing (within mental health work, generally) sometimes subverts the debate about professionalism, nevertheless, it is deeply entrenched in existing definitions and as part of the purchaser driven ethos of contemporary nursing practice.

Political skills do not form part of the nursing criteria at pre or post registration level. Nursing seems to be apolitical without possessing the relevant leadership to bring politics into the nursing arena. Even in mental health, where nurses have a less prissy and more militant image, it is often argued that nursing is defined by a different value and belief system, one that always considers the patient first and the political agenda of nursing second. Bearing this in mind, it is not surprising that political issues in small child and adolescent services are usually taken with those of psychiatry as a whole. Further analysis reveals nursing's historical lack of influence and political clout in the key health policy decision-making processes that, ultimately, affect patient outcomes. This has been attributed to the unconfident, deferential, and hierarchical behaviour of nurses and the traditional inability of nursing to find a unified political objective. The nursing professions deliver 80% of direct care (Beardshaw and Robinson, 1990), yet have little or no representation within the wider political domain. Nurses collectively play rather little part in local or regional political activity, apart from joining the occasional RCN conference when they can jeer at a scapegoat speaker. To this end, there has been, to date, little work undertaken that systematically examines the effect on current changes in health care of politically-involved nurses. One change will be the long awaited recognition of nursing as a full profession. However, this desire for professional status among nurses reflects their weakness in the politics of health care. This is shown by the evident gap between the rhetoric of nursing and the reality of its practice, which is dominated by the medical and managerial cultures (Kubsch, 1996).

Nursing is as much a prisoner of powerful psychiatry as the young people who are held within psychiatry's diagnostic criteria. A criteria, as noted by our friendly critic Pursey, 'which purports to give answers to psychological deviance'. The power of psychiatry stems from the higher social status of medicine, i.e. a profession that is largely self-employed, self-regulating and still accorded a respect (for its views) that goes largely unchallenged. That is what gives the DSM book its magic power: I say you're ill, because I'm a doctor. The nurse may modify the diagnosis or even challenge it. The doctor may gracefully alter judgement, but the nurse's views only make sense in the context of a doctor (ultimately) underwriting them. However, as long as psychiatry possesses the magic book of diagnostic classification, it will always possess and process the power, one that is employed and exercised through a net-like organisation (Richer, 1990). Both ideology and power exist irrespective of individuals. In a similar vein, Habermas (1971) holds that there is no end for ideology, Richer (1990) notes how Foucault's (1980) position regarding power is anti-subjectivist, arguing that 'individuals or classes are the vehicles of power, not its source'. The use of diagnostic criteria is acknowledged as being one of the major conflicts within the psychiatric care of mentally ill young people. It must be argued daily by nurses in the majority of ward rounds and patient reviews that psychiatrists insist upon labelling and falsely diagnosing young people, irrespective of the evidence placed before them, like some gift from a servant. We hardly need the suspicious postmodern emphasis on viewing the theoretical surface of 'what seems to be' to discover that one does not have to scratch very hard in order to discover oppositions, irregularities and hidden assumptions beneath our daily practice. Nursing has a servant-like role. Yet we still continue to maintain the boundaries of practice because of our fear of a breakdown in the neatly conceptualised frameworks already in place. In fact, nursing has gone one step further in a splendid attempt to be even more modernist than the hand that feeds it. The use of a nursing process and nursing diagnostic criteria are two important examples of how nursing has attempted to undermine the power base of psychiatry at the expense of the patient, as the price of attaining professional modernity.

The ideology of the nursing process

Institutions have been justified in terms of providing safety to the mentally ill, disordered, and 'rebellious youth of today'. We, the authors, argue that the provision of Tier 4 services has been promoted by a modern preoccupation with madness and the supposedly legitimate classification or diagnosis of mental illness. To this end, this chapter aims to be post modern in flavour and content. Other nursing text books on child and adolescent mental health (or should we say psychiatry?) base their entire epistemology upon the diagnostic and subsequent treatment modalities of mental illness. It is often with great pride that second editions provide a revised chapter on the ever more elaborate taxonomy of childhood diagnosis. This book has resisted the temptation to provide a regular classification of medical terms, such as conduct disorder, emotional regressive disorder, and attachment deficits and offers, instead, a broader, more complex approach that we know is harder to synthesise, but one that continues to open the debate relevant to child and adolescent issues that the HAS Report (1995) has already begun. The problems of labelling, and the defeatist tendency of conceding that even a 'scientifically objective' diagnostic system is better than no system at all, have to be challenged. We are not crudely anti-medical, but we are deeply sceptical of the claims of 'scientific' psychiatry, as are many others. We aim to offer an alternative world-view for nurses caring for young people's mental health.

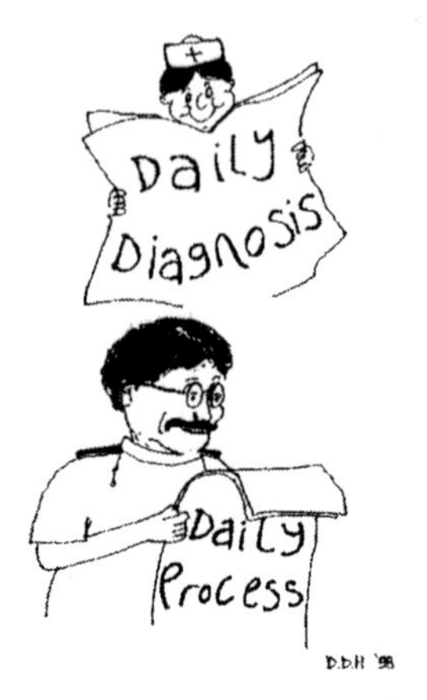

The nursing process

The development of nursing as a process finds its roots in the nursing models of the 1950s and 1960s. The aim of systematising care, flattening skill mix, and providing a theoretical base from which a fledgling profession could proudly emerge has resulted in a standardised framework that is now part of the fabric of nursing. According to Benner and Wrubel (1989), the majority of current nursing theories are in the tradition of classical science and, as such, maintain that a human being, like the universe, can be considered machine-like, orderly, predictable, observable, and measurable. Paterson and Zderad (1988) feel that mechanistic scientific theory-building is not fully able to express the complexity of the aesthetic qualities of the nature of nursing practice.

Assessment

It is assumed that assessment in the context of the nursing process is about collecting, gathering, and storing information about a young person. This is either directly by questioning, interviews, and questionnaires, or less direct methods, such as observation. The process is continuous throughout the work performed by the nurse and young person, and forms an integral part of the relationship. The process of assessing young people belongs within a framework of conceptual theory, which usually involves the nursing team contemplating the effective or ineffective functioning of the young person. The facets of this functioning can be reduced further to specific behaviours, mood, interaction, language, etc. Other methods of assessment include the retrospective examination of patient records and consultation with parents and significant others.

According to research, agreement between parents and young people tends to be very limited, as noted by Costello (1986). Findings seem to be common to all assessment methods, that is, checklists and questionnaires, and to data collected by interview. One solution utilised widely in community settings by nurse specialists is to interview young people and parents serially. This involves always interviewing the young person first to promote an alliance and then, if possible, immediately interviewing the parents in the company of the young person. By doing this, any issues raised can be dealt with immediately. The combination of checklist and interview seems to be a the most useful method to elicit assessment data.

Diagnosis

Broadly speaking, nursing diagnosis is the first process in analysing and constructing a meaning from the information obtained from the assessment. As noted by Bellack and Edlund (1992: 9) 'Nursing diagnoses are a client's responses to actual or potential health problems, not the health problems themselves'. Tentative diagnostic hypotheses (inferences) are developed and then confirmation sought. Castledine (1991b) makes reference to the diagnostic component of advanced practice. The ability to diagnose has a direct relationship with being an expert. As noted by Calkin (1984), 'Nurses who excel in analysis and insight when diagnosing and treating human responses are generally known as experts'.

The nursing diagnosis of ill young people is asking questions, such as: 'What is wrong here; What are the current responses to interaction, illness, health; What are the effects of family visits?' In order to support diagnostic formulations within the framework of the nursing process, the ability to critically reason or think about patients' underlying attitudes and beliefs, which may be supporting illness-related behaviours, enables nurses to provide an answer to: 'How do we provide appropriate action to progress towards health?' Therefore, critical thinking is a cognitive process, an ability that encompasses maturity and inquisitiveness. It is an ability that seems to improve with experience and practice; however, critical thinking means questioning personal practice, as discussed in Benner's (1984) model of skill acquisition. It involves the dominant ideology of reflective practice and the formulation of abstract conceptualisations in 'deciding what to believe or do' (Kataoka-Yahiro and Saylor, 1994). Hence, the 'novice' nurse will more than likely be very proficient at doing 'nursing by the book'. Perhaps our 'novice's book will be similar to other books on child and adolescent units, which describe the members of the MDT, and the routines one might expect and the behaviours exhibited by certain illness categorisations. The novice's learning will be part of the critical thinking process. As skills and exposure increase, more information is available for abstracting and testing. The nurse may begin to formulate personal hypotheses about the nature of the care young people receive, but it is not until a multitude of factors have been processed (including position in the hierarchy and the development of a personal supportive network) that most critical thinking can be put into action for directly changing patient care.

Historical development of nursing diagnosis

It seems that nursing diagnosis is not a new phenomenon; rather, it has been pointedly neglected for a number of reasons. Theoretically, it originally belonged as the second component of the nursing process, e.g. Assessment, Diagnosis, Planning, Implementation, Evaluation. However, for whatever reasons, it was not favoured by medics who suspected an encroachment into their diagnostic domain or by nurse theorists who sought to objectify nursing on a similar modernist model. As noted by Hogston (1997), 'Nursing diagnosis originated in North America in the 1970s in an effort to move the art, science, and theoretical basis of nursing forward'. The North American Nursing Diagnosis Association (NANDA, 1990) has promoted the development of nursing diagnosis in the USA. The American Nurses Association (ANA), in its standards of practice, defined nursing as 'the diagnosis and treatment of human responses to actual or potential health problems' (Carpenito, 1995: 5, cited in Hogston).

In the UK, it seems that nursing diagnosis as an integral part of a nursing process is neglected. It has been suggested that the language and conceptual framework adopted by NANDA is abstract and not easily understood by British nurses (Hogston, 1997). However, it can be argued that, for nurses in the UK, the use of systems approach to nursing indirectly utilises diagnostic tools and skills in order to hypothesise 'patient problems' and mode of nursing intervention. It could be suggested that the exchange of 'problem' for diagnosis would be a feasible operation to permit the development of a British nursing diagnostic base. However, this ignores the fact that, as a process, there is a need for a solid epistemology to guide practice. Therefore, just substituting labels will not be enough. Also, as noted by Alexander *et al* (1995), most British nursing care plans are focussed upon medical diagnosis. This seems to have implications for what is emerging as the new professionalism, as nursing strives to rid itself of its traditional 'handmaiden image'. The use of language and common terminology is used to promote an elitism that secures professional power and, we believe, excludes the young people we treat from the planning of their care. The care process will become more reductionist and, therefore, more oppressive if nursing diagnosis becomes more prevalent within the nursing process.

Concluding remarks

As community care and trust economics progress, it seems that the selling of expertness will become second nature within the contemporary health trade. Perhaps liaison mental health nursing has the 'potential to shape the future delivery of nursing care and to identify new and evolving specialisms', such as links with accident and emergency units, health visitors, and other non-mental health services. Such a development would require the ANP (advanced nurse practitioner) to conduct assessments and manage a programme- centred approach outside the traditional culture of the mental health setting. The important concept of nurse consultation is tightly linked to improved nursing knowledge, to richer, non-medical modes of nursing diagnosis and, of course, to an expansion of the role of nurses. That expansion would have to be politically defended, as having economical advantages and as advancing patient-centred care. The aim then, is to be able to justify nursing expansion. To do this, it is necessary to have a science of nursing to justify practice. Science as well as art is an important weapon within nursing ideology, which can be successfully exploited. In North America, this process is reflected in the way science is cast against humanism and hermeneutics. 'Hermeneutical understanding can enlighten the human state (Gortner, 1990). This is also reflected in the increasing momentum of an increased academic commitment. The past decade has witnessed momentous political and organisational change in the NHS, fundamental changes in basic nurse education and the post basic education now necessary for periodic registration. These have all contributed to the development of a professional nursing ethos.

Nursing diagnostic taxonomies provide frameworks for the diagnosis of young people's problems and help in (as noted by Hogston (1997)) 'advancing the professional status of nursing'. The idea of nursing diagnosis is one that may fill many with dread, because classification is anti-holist and pigeon-holes young people. However, as a method for expanding practice, nursing diagnosis is, according to Lutzen and Tishelman, (1996) (cited in Hogston), a method of defining and organising nursing care. This ultimately gives nursing a unique platform upon which professionalism is more secure. As a tool, it is more concerned with pattern recognition, where previous exposure to a particular illness, interaction, or incident allows more options for guiding the nurse's work. This means it is young person-led, rather than being used to provide labels as in medical diagnosis.

Chapter 5
Modern manufacturing: ideology, culture and assumptions

The rich man in his castle,
The poor man at his gate,
He made them high and lowly,
And ordered their estate.

All things bright and beautiful ...

Cecil Frances Alexander (1823–1895)

Dialogue

Sandy: Has it occurred to you how often nursing is seen as an industry, you know...as belonging to the twentieth century ethos of production?

Dean: You mean like a work force producing health, etc?

Sandy: Sort of. Think about it. Nursing belongs to a historical culture that ultimately reflects the wider nature of society. Nursing has adopted an industrial 'Fordism' complete with production lines. Most of the arguments regarding the application of theoretical models centre around a limited number, which seem to reinforce the dominant ideology and cultures of nursing.

Dean: You mean behaviourism and systems theory are the tools of our trade; they virtually define the boundaries of our remit?

Sandy: Not only that, we should decide how important it is to recognise that nursing ideology and culture has an impact on what we do as nurses, and then locate the dominant care models, such as behaviourism, etc.

Dean: I think it would be easier just to give a description of each theory and model like other books have done.

Sandy: But is it relevant if we are re-thinking about the effects of (M)odernity? Because ideology and culture are formed, and are part of the large structures that determine practice, regardless of individual agency.

Dean: What ever you say...I'm just a manufactured product of my time and culture and not an 'agency' nurse.

Thesis for this chapter

- ❑ Power and ideology are major concerns of postmodernist philosophy
- ❑ Technology and progress are ideological constructs in that, as nurses, our knowledge has validity and meaning only in terms of the latest technology we subscribe to
- ❑ Technologies are assumed to be somehow linked to scientific discovery for their legitimation. For example, nurses will often defend pychodynamic theory as being grounded in scientific research and reason.

Background and aims

All Tier 4 residential units (as with community services) have living active cultures. It is also usual to assume that there are always sub-cultures that are dependant upon a dominant culture. There are many definitions as to what culture actually is, but it is usually assumed that culture is based upon tradition; our profession has been built upon generations of nursing practice, which helps sustain the status quo, acts as a containing force, and prevents erosion of the dominant ideology. The ideology is based upon wider beliefs about the four core concepts of nursing: the environment, man/behaviour, nursing, and health. As such, the culture of every unit is moulded by mixtures of socio-cultural, milieu, and behaviour theories together with various models that include: functionalism, psycho-cultural systems, and communications models. The *staff* world is one that has to be negotiated and learned by all new staff and learners. So, although all unit cultures have their own peculiar slants, there are common core concepts that appear repeatedly. These include: issues of power, hierarchy, compliance, competition, leadership, motivation cycles, the favourite patient, discipline, work control, social support—the list goes on and on. This chapter aims to explore these issues of the staff world of institutional care of children and adolescents.

Aims:

1. To provide brief descriptions of the dominant technologies (theories) which rationalise notions of progress, expertness, and power/knowledge. These are: behaviour theory, socio-cultural theories, and grand systems theory;

2. To explore the issue of ideology, science, and technology in relation to the dominant discourses in psychiatric belief and assumptions;
3. To explore the common core concepts of power hierarchy, leadership, and ideology in relation to organisational structure.

Introduction

Most work on the study of cultures, beliefs, and assumptions is of a sociological nature and, therefore, a (M)odern phenomenon, e.g., the work of Goffman, Mead. The concept of a progressive culture is closely interwoven with the values embraced by a community. It is a deep structure that finds expression in people's knowledge, beliefs, convictions, morals, and laws. Various adjectives can be attached to culture: popular, high, elite, Western. As such, past events and anticipation for the future are all reflected in culture. For the authors, culture in its simplest framework can be viewed as a system of learned and shared standards for perceiving, interpreting, and behaving in interactions with others and the environment. This shares the tradition of Goffmanian sociology (Goffman, 1961) and of Sartre (1992) by seeking to explore existential and constructivist aspects of social life. Regarding the agency individual nurses are able to utilise with children and young people, it is possible to refer to a dynamic tension that focusses debate upon the nature of health care provision, dependent upon the political ideology of the times, and the socio-economic circumstances. In Neo-Marxist theory— particularly that of the Frankfurt school—the growth of mass consumption, commodities, and competitive markets is intrinsically linked to the persistence of exploitative ideology; for example, the dominant theories of human science are used to justify unequal relations of production. In our case, the production of beneficial health outcomes or, seen from another perspective, the labelling and insertion of a youngster into Tier 4 service provision; the dominant view of illness produces another young person adapted to the sick role. Professionals' false consciousness results from nurses, first, tolerating an inferior position within NHS super structures and, second, having only a limited choice of theoretical models of practice. Nurses are constantly under pressure and expected to make choices regarding the nature of their practice and the models they adopt. Their understanding and demonstration of these limited pseudo-sciences is seen as a standard of practice (nowadays reflective practice) and ability to attain promotion.

This chapter aims to answer the question: To what extent does a nurse have any say over the way she practices? Prior to discussing this in detail, it is necessary to highlight the dominant theories used by nurses working with children and young people, in order to demonstrate that a nurse's agency, her ability to act with a conscious sense of autonomy and independence, is determined by a limited choice of considered or preferred models that are radically different in the propositions they advance. As noted by Kvale (1990: 9), postmodernist authors who draw upon Foucault's analysis of the inter-penetration of knowledge and power in the social sciences see the political implications of postmodernism as leading not to apathy, but to activism. In the same way, Masson (1990) and Richer (1990) deconstruct modern humanistic and therapeutic psychology, and attack them as techni-quasi forms of oppression. It is worth reflecting upon the sentiments of Richer (1990), who sees all psychology as partaking in (M)odernity's categorising and clarifying human behaviour, and having a police role, with psychodynamic and humanist psychology, as the secret police. This reminds us of the call by Lather (1990; 101) in earlier chapters to deconstruct humanist philosophy to reveal the nature of relationships within written language, and the social relationships young people have in leading the good life towards others. At its most cynical, this can translate to 'following the rules of the unit' and 'the rules of society', regardless of what autonomy you have.

Dominant theories that rationalise nursing practice

Behaviour theory

Behaviourism is synonymous with the twentieth century and goes in and out of vogue as cultural shifts occur. It is prominent in public policy discussions about treating delinquency, from the political footballs of 'boot camps' and capital punishment, to smacking a child when he is naughty. Of course, it is now politically incorrect to condone corporal punishments. The state has intervened in that domain, which, not too long ago, was the sphere of the individual. As such, the legal embodiment of the rights of children (The Children Act, 1989) attempts to uphold politically correct standards to empower both children and carers, with guidelines that are anti-behavioural and appeal to the more interpersonal theories. However, behaviourism has a large audience who take easily observed events, such as destructiveness, violence, and anti-socialness, as being evidence for the failure of 'wishy- washy do-gooding'.

Behaviourist theory, with its biological basis, has contributed a lot to theories of motivation in nursing. It is philosophically deterministic and the implementation of operant conditioning techniques of positive and negative reinforcement has been a mainstay for nurses working with children, usually in the pursuit of extinguishing unwanted behaviour. Learning theorists propose that many neurotic and psychotic symptoms seen in childhood are not necessarily the result of developmental difficulties, but rather the result of learned, but unadaptive behavioural patterns that are maintained by their consequences; for example, attention of adults and lots of exciting uproar. It is a central premise that all behaviour is learned and so, therefore, can be unlearned and re-taught. This is usually implemented using behaviour modification techniques, practice, and reinforcement of rewards. Desensitisation, assertiveness training, role play, and advise-giving all fall within the spectrum of behaviour modification, and are used extensively by child and adolescent nurses daily. It is common to see behavioural care plans in many adolescent units, even if the underlying culture is one that promotes systems theory, or more psychodynamic techniques of practice. It is futile to separate 'behaviour' (of a young patient) from who the patient is, or from what he/she presently believes. Of course behaviour is a key part of how we experience and assess our patients, whatever our philosophical perspective as nurses. However, all too often, children are equated with their behaviour, as if they consisted in it, as if according to Pursey (friendly critic), they were confined to it. As a result, they, and our ability to help them, may come to be confined by their behaviour. Similarly, the way a nurse implements care is viewed by his/her colleagues through his/her actions in specific interactions.

The history of behaviourism, its use to human society, and its underlying philosophy in its modern application sense can be, at least in part, traced back to Fredrick Wilson Taylor (1856-1915). He was concerned with the efficiency and effectiveness of a modern day work force as a functioning unit in a capitalist enterprise, as opposed to a collection of individuals. In a way, nursing has experienced the consequences of Taylorism. Taylor's belief was that both parties within a capitalist work force, the employer and the employee, have a common interest and a common measurable goal of efficiency in production. Although highly criticised in its early days (and now), such crude human engineering was adopted as a profitable modern model of 'production', and this can certainly be seen in the often quoted primary nurse and task allocation systems popular in nursing. The behaviourist J B Watson, in his early career, worked closely with industry and he, like the growing number of psychologists, was interested in the evolutionary aspects of industry. His concern, as noted by Smith (1997: 609), involved developing 'new technologies and knowledge as the means to carry human evolution forward'; as such, his polemical view has as 'its theoretical goal... the prediction and control of behaviour'.

The study of behaviour, in particular the notions of motivation, adaption, and adjustment, symbolised an evolutionary attempt to understand the significance of modern social arrangements upon individual actors. Prior to this century, such work was limited. In the first six decades of the twentieth century, behaviourism focussed on what it could do for society and (as will be discussed shortly) functionalist theory provided the pragmatic vehicle and approach through which behaviourism could be legitimised, as an evolutionary breakthrough in understanding the individual in modern society. All of this has had dramatic consequences for the care of young people during the closing decades of this century, because the positivist epistemology of behaviourism has supported its claim of legitimacy in a scientific world view. Behavioural science will include the human in its studies as one organism among many; in this, it apes the objectivity of the natural scientist studying nature. Similarly, behaviourism dismisses the problem of meaning (the so called black box notion) because, as Watson (1983) argued, 'We watch what the animal or human being is doing. He 'means' what he 'does'.' The popular guide, Psychological Care of Infant and Child (Watson and Rayner, 1920), emphasised this notion and also heralded the arrival of psychology into the arena of child rearing, parenting, and child development. Similarly, the work of Melanie Klein, and Anna Freud in the psychodynamic and psychoanalytic fields of psychology reflected the growing popularity of the, supposedly, progressive science of psychology, which quickly became part of the modern citizen's commonsense view of the world. Psychology, legitimised as a science, became available as a care and saviour of 'lost' children, a bridge between the unknown parts of a child's psyche and the rational, trainable, assessable, and (M)odern parts. This also had consequences for the child of the latter twentieth century, because the myth that modern society has created a new and devastating illness, as well as the existing natural or biological ones, legitimised the continued existence of positivist psychology and psychiatry. This 'problem of ideology' will also be discussed later during this chapter.

The Vienna group of philosophers in the 1930s shared the same distaste for metaphysics as that shown by believers in behaviourism and functionalism. The effect of this age of empirically grounded theory, prior to the second world war, was to embed the notion that there is a single observable and empirically verifiable form of science. In short, the subjective was meaningless, the objective was truth. Thus, the philosophical foundations of behaviourism belong to the positivist framework favoured throughout modern psychiatry's 100-year history. The development of holistic and eclectic models allow for behaviourism's inclusion as a valid and substantial contribution in all nursing and psychiatric assessment. The formality of observing and recording objective behaviour is based upon an epistemology, which insists that the natural and human world can be described in terms of a systematic theory based on observed facts and deduction. The neo-behaviourism offered by Skinner's operant psychology emphasises behaviourism's obsession with the observable and, therefore, the body as behaviour. This can be likened to the psychiatric 'gaze' discussed by Foucault (1971), which is an idea that will be discussed in the third section of this book in more detail. According to Skinner (1953), behaviour included thought and language (which is one of the major concerns of postmodernist thinkers); language and thought being, to Skinner, just another form of learned behaviour. Clearly, this denies the notion of freewill and takes away individual responsibility. In such a context, survival or existence is a fact not a value, whether we consider individuals or society. However, it is values and assumptions that we, as nurses, make about the young people we nurse that affects the care they experience. As noted by Smith (1997: 672), behaviourism 'and other natural sciences did not satisfactorily deal with values'. Therefore, behaviourism (being probably mostly used in the care of young people as opposed to adults) is underpinned by ideology in the form of functionalist theory. So, this apparently pragmatic and practical method is widely utilised in nursing young people today.

Functionalism model

The human sciences of functional explanation are rooted in evolutionary, holistic, and determinist philosophy. Functional explanation attempts to apply biological concepts to the macro nature of human society and organisation. The model proposes that society is an organic whole, which is continuously in a state of flux. Functionalists, like Durkheim, Merton and Parsons, emphasised that institutions and various groups in society are needed to ensure that the whole runs smoothly, thus maintaining equilibrium. As noted by Pasquali *et al* (1989), 'new ideas and practices that maintain the existing social order are readily accepted by members of society', but 'Ideas and practices which seriously disrupt the existing social order tend to be resisted'. From this, there begins to appear similarities with most ward cultures. The idea of 'law and order' is reflected in hierarchy and the need for legitimacy in authority. Power maintains the *status quo* in order to maintain the smooth functioning of the entire system. As a group, individuals within society have to live by certain rules, values, and standards; inpatient units, containing a microcosm of society, are often thought to be societies in themselves.

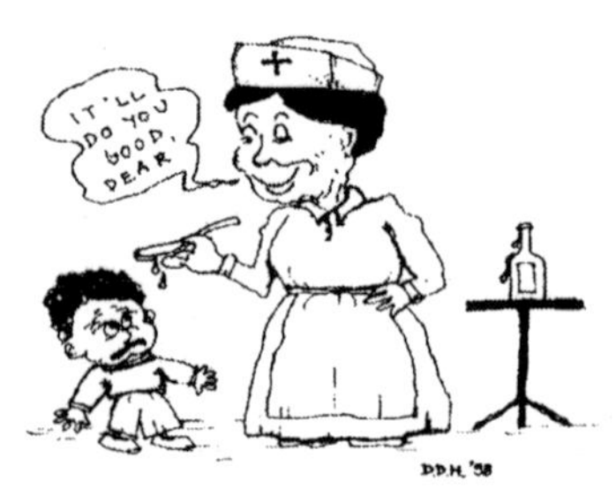

Imagine the expectations placed upon the first adolescent units of the 1950s and 1960s. The standard belief was that society functioned like nature and that ill young people who were inefficient needed to be removed, repaired, and then replaced as functioning wholes back into a nuclear family unit, which itself was efficient. Such removing bore witness to the lingering superstition that mental illness was infectious: removal, therefore, would prevent an epidemic of unknown natural illness among civilised man. The progressive vision of functionalism symbolised both behaviourism's and functionalism's ability to sustain an ideology of understanding human nature and the nature of mental illness, and provide some protection from the latter. As noted by Smith (1997: 484), 'Political values support the view that the activity of the parts of society should be understood in terms of the contribution of the parts to the economic efficiency of the whole'. As such, the functionalist emphasis on measuring appeared to offer a solution to understanding man in relation to society. Such solutions only comprise those which can be observed and objectively accounted for.

The concern to account for what young people 'do' rather than what they think formalised its position as a dominant way of thinking. From it arose practices, like the use of boot camps, discipline, and behavioural rewards to young people in trouble with society at large.

The psychocultural model focusses upon the relationship between the individual psyche and the social field (Pasquali *et al*, 1989). The development of children is specifically well suited in terms of these models of personality development. Infants are exposed to the family unit or other significant carers and from here develop and experience society. Society is a strange place in which they have to attach and form meaningful relationships with teachers, other family members, siblings, peers, and other socialising agents. Society exposes them to hierarchy, manners, expectations, norms, and values of society. 'Don't be cheeky and rude', 'It was very good of you to help Jonathan with his shoe laces'. Once again the deterministic nature of this model expects that most children will reach and pass through set developmental milestones, as they learn to curb their inner desires and wants in favour of that which is expected of them. They learn their position in the wider world and the sanctions that will keep order. The simplistic appearance of fixed causation between moral actions and consequences gave functionalism advantages as a system of thought against the subjective thought beginning to gain ground in continental Europe.

The dominant theories, which rationalise the nursing care of young people, are the adopted technology that is supposed to advancing nursing per se as a science and art. A number of questions arise from an analysis of their use. How do we account for their differences? Why have some models made greater or more rapid impact in the treatment of children and adolescents than, say, the now emerging post-modernist/constructivist explanations of human relationships? What was the stimulus for such supposed technological advances? Why have hypnotherapy, reflexology, and acupuncture remained on the fringes, compared to client-centred humanistic eclectic psychotherapy, cognitive behavioural therapy, behaviourism, and systems theory? Did these technologies set the pace for political and social change or were these developments a product of economic, ideological, and cultural status? In order to begin unpicking the general assumptions behind the answers to these and many other questions, it is necessary to consider the ideological framework within which they developed. In particular, the modern assumptions beginning to be uncovered in this book: 'ideas of progress', 'the triumph of rationality and logic', 'the quest for a distinct nursing knowledge base', 'enclosed boundaries of nursing practice', 'caring as a core facet to practice', and 'child-centeredness'.

Nursing ideology

According to Williams (1976), ideology can be thought of as being 'abstract thought'. It concerns speculative systems, which themselves belong to the metaphysics and discourses of the twentieth century. Abercrombie *et al* (1984) further defines ideology as beliefs, attitudes and opinions that are bound together, either loosely or very tightly. Thus, there appear to be two main schools of thought regarding ideology. First, there are those who consider ideology to be mostly neutral, such as Thompson (1986: 24), who argues that ideologies reproduce 'the social order by symbolically representing it as a unity in which the individual has a place' (Taylor, 1997). Second, the majority of writers present ideology in a critical modernist sense, that is, from the perspective of moral or political philosophy. For Marx, ideology was reductionist—everything could eventually be reduced to economic terms, and his ideology assumes that there is opposition between appearance and reality. Ideology is a means of maintaining power at the expense of those with less power (Giddens, 1993; cited in Taylor, 1997).

The dominant ideology of British nursing encompasses concepts of humanism and holism that centre on the nurse-child relationship (Rafferty, 1991). As such, when combined with the acceptable face of a positive, if somewhat altruistic ideology embodied in the notion of child centeredness, it is easy to assume that nursing ideology has the young person at heart. However, this is not necessarily the case, as power relationships always have one individual with more power than the other at the micro/interactional level. It is usually the child or young person with less power. This can be seen in the general assumptions nurses have about nursing mentally ill young people. Their assumptions are ideologically loaded and based upon metaphysical contradictions that are very rarely questioned. Although it is not possible or even desirable to change the caring assumptions that accumulate in nursing ideology, it is important to acknowledge their presence in order to create informed practice. Therefore, the issue of power is an important concept to understand.

General assumptions of nursing young people.

- ❑ That young people in hospital are there because they need to be
- ❑ That young people in hospital would be nursed in the community if possible
- ❑ Preventative nursing is better than crisis intervention
- ❑ Caring for the young people is the most important thing
- ❑ Medication should be used if necessary
- ❑ All young people and children should be nursed as individuals with unique care needs
- ❑ The nurse-young person relationship attempts to alleviate power issues
- ❑ Young people belong to a wider world
- ❑ Power comes from within
- ❑ In order to alleviate mental distress, it is important to talk
- ❑ Some young people need expert help to ensure they attain mental health
- ❑ Mental illness exists, so does mental health
- ❑ The individual is the unit of society
- ❑ Individual young people are a product of their nature
- ❑ Individual young people are a product of their environment
- ❑ Individual young people are a product of their upbringing
- ❑ Treat physical needs first
- ❑ Having a knowledge of psychology means you can read people's minds.

Figure 5.1: Satirising of the commonsense model

Ideology as an industry

Ideology has the role of ordering hierarchy and maintaining the *status quo*; and, in nursing, it shadows the political and industrial power structures. Psychiatry as a body of political and scientific knowledge (and in its relationship to society) has the dominance to determine which technologies prevail and how they are regulated, and guarantee the environment in which technology develops. As regulator, it sets standards for how technology affects the everyday life of professionals and young people alike. The 'scientific management of Taylor (1911) is reflected in the nursing process as a way of structuring nursing activity

(What have you got to do this shift nurse?). This ideological ordering is seen as providing the best product for those who require it, deserve it, and have a right to it. Nursing is no longer a career that is standardised against the backdrop of caring alone. Consumerism is a paradoxical ingredient in a free-market enterprise (Jones, 1994) and, as such, belongs to modern times with modern demands and expected standards. It involves a process of social evolution towards higher expectations, similar to those experienced in all other walks of life. Everything has to be disposable, plastic, quick, efficient, and well worth the money. Such a market place is a socially-constructed entity rather than a naturally occurring one. And, as such, the market brings with it a diverse mixture of differences, in professional language, status, and mechanisms of production. These are mechanisms that permit conspiracy between competing professional groups. The situation is that the more powerful groups dominate the very ideas and thought processes that frame health care. 'Production' is organised and maintained by both the management bureaucrat and the strongest male-dominated professional group—medicine. As noted by Hopton (1997), 'psychiatrists require nurses to keep their patients under surveillance in order to confirm their diagnosis and to administer and monitor the treatments they prescribe'. As such, nursing is the production line, as well as the departments of maintenance and quality inspection. The behavioural, sociocultural, and systems theories previously discussed are the tools of the trade, which keep the machinery moving.

As noted by Hilton (1997), most representations of nursing reflect the view that nursing is concerned with managing the interaction between the child and the environment to promote health and well being. Nursing activity consists of regulating, promoting, modifying, maintaining, and monitoring the interaction between the patient and the environment, and also maintaining communication and social interaction. The usual displays of power relate to the way a nurse is able to demonstrate authority and be perceived as being more powerful than the child. More subtle ways include the way interaction is regulated in the context of what is supposedly beneficial to the young person. Nurses are experienced in this type of shop floor policing. It reflects the power and the historical prerogative nursing has over the daily activities of young hospitalised patients. This carries the sentiment of both Hilton (1997) and Therborn (1980) that nursing ideologies are legitimised by tradition, a reliance on medicine, and unequal power. Such ideology also legitimises the development of nursing cultures, which have an effect on both young people and the nurses who care for them. The notions of effectiveness, efficiency, and technological progress are our common ideological currency. The ideological framework of psychiatry determines how technologies prevail. Technologies, such as, behaviourism, socio-cultural theories, or functionalism have no special logic or momentum of their own. Their value and the assumptions—be they right or wrong—made from them, and other technologies, reflect the wider intellectual arena in which desired technological standards are assumed. These assumptions guide and shape their adaption, adoption, and success or failure. The way this is done is termed 'the problem of ideology' (Moore, 1989: 30). Nursing ideology, as a system of interrelated ideas, assumptions and the afore-mentioned desires, therefore, misrepresents the reality of the young people that it claims is central to practice.

As also noted by Moore, an ideology or belief is said to be ideological because 'it participates in an ideology that offers a subjective, over simplified, partial, abnormal, distorted unscientific, or just plain uncommonsensical view of the world'. In this respect, ideology is ideological and so is this book. This is not shameful, but to ignore the ideological frameworks inherent to nursing might well be. Ideology of child and adolescent mental health nursing is a view of the world from the standpoint of a powerful, dominating interested party: psychiatry. It categorises the experience of young people, interprets their activities and the boundaries they make between concepts, such as, different technological therapeutic models, relationships, diagnosis, and separate spheres of role. This has been a main ideological assertion throughout this book. The technology nursing uses gives rise to ideology in ordinary practice. This ideology, in turn, as noted by Moore, serves to justify or legitimate technology. This notion of legitimacy, which has been a recurring theme, is a piece of heuristic reasoning related to how nurses experience their everyday practice. The belief that technology will find solutions to the difficulties experienced by young people is legitimised by ideology, an ideology that is a modernist myth. One example to consider is the anxious parents who take their oddly behaving child to an expert to receive the psychotherapy they've heard about on TV.

(M)odernist dogma holds that all problems, whether natural, cultural, or social, can be cured by technology or the continued development of it for future generations. The difficulty arises when we consider the values associated with the separating of purely pragmatic solutions made by technology, and the outcomes experienced by the young person. These ethical dilemmas, faced by nurses each and everyday, are made tolerable by the ideological and cultural belief that we give the best that is known at present. The emphasis that the technology we employ is neutral is a myth. The technology is intrinsically linked to the culture served by nursing. According to Layton (1977), no one model of the relations of science, technology, and society is entailed by a standard science/technology dichotomy, but it is certainly compatible with the simplest, so-called linear sequential models of technical innovations, in which technology sits in the middle, developing innovations spun off pure scientific research, and tailoring them to the demands of the public and private sectors of the economy (Chant, 1989). The idea that the science of nursing as an ideology of progressive technology is somehow an exalted pursuit of truth is a myth. Although both Popper and Kuhn have, in different ways, undermined this positivist view of science as the progressive unfolding of truth, according to Chant (1989), neither subscribes to the opposite (and postmodern) view, the claim that scientific truth is relative only to the culture in which scientists practice. The technology used to take care of many mentally ill young people shares in the ideological and cultural assumptions of society at large, including one held by many practitioners—namely, a belief in technological determinism.

Technological determinism

Philosophically speaking, determinism is a notion that every event has a natural cause, or, as noted by Chant (1989: 48), is the (in principle) predictable outcome of the operation of natural laws—a position frequently associated with the ethically significant rejection of free will or freedom of choice. Therefore, technological determinism (as a notion that all social and cultural change is ultimately dependant upon technological change and vis versa) provides the authors with a troublesome thesis, one suggesting that nurses, as with other MDT professionals caring for mentally ill young people, are not necessarily autonomous practitioners, but rather they are reliant upon the technology available to them at their given time in any given culture. Such a controversial proposition can be seen to mirror Marx's materialist conception of history: critical theory or critique of advanced capitalism, identified by the Frankfurt School, is usually associated with Marx. Chant (1989: 49) offers a succinct overview of historical materialism, which describes a sequence of historical events in which changes in the 'forces of production' determined the 'social relations of production'; these, in turn, decided all social relations, in particular the dimensions of social classes. From this position, it is possible to reflect upon the work of Marcuse, who was influenced by a humanist rather than a technocist reading of Marx, which, according to Chant (p52), enabled Marcuse to reflect upon the power and even beneficence of modern technology, especially its part in a growing fetishism of commodities. We can identify commodities in mental health nursing in topics, such as, client-centred approaches, medications and reflective practice and, more recently, supervision, CPA, and active outreach.

Legitimisation

Ideology might be operationalised by legitimisation. Legitimisation is based on the grounds of rationality, tradition, and charisma. The Code of Professional Conduct (United Kingdom Central Council for Nursing, Midwifery, and Health Visiting, 1992) exemplifies this, and nurses are accustomed to feel secure with a set of rules to obey. Nursing is extremely traditional. There is usually a strong chain of command, lubricated by fear. Thompson (1990) expands on Weber's legitimisation—strategies employed in nursing include: rationalisation, universalisation, and fragmentation. We would add patientisation (Taylor, 1997). Rationalisation is a chain of reasoning that seeks to justify actions. Universalisation is a tool used in legitimating the nursing ideology. 'The subordinate group learns to internalise its subordination and it becomes part of their collective personality' (Ford and Walsh, 1994: 45). Political, managerial, and nursing agendas can all be disguised as being in the patient's interest. Thus British idealism and taste for collective responsibility in health was enshrined in four basic principles: meeting needs, equity, access to the best service, and containment of health costs. Similarly, ideology and science are often contrasted as alternative ways of representing knowledge of the world. Scientific argument is said to be based on evidence and truth, while ideological argument is based on values and beliefs. While science has a major role to play in nursing practice, the total world view of nursing can only be represented as an ideology. The most important feature of ideology is not whether it is true, but whether it is successful (Rushing, 1993).

Career hierarchies of specialised occupations (not all equal in status or reward) characterise the modern work place. As noted by our friendly critic, Pursey, the idea of professionalism also attracts because it gives a sense of belonging to a supra-group, transcending the conditions of an alienating and hostile workplace. New practitioners are inducted 'into a mystery' complete with one's unique role. Professionalism centres on a specialised knowledge, expertise, education, service, autonomy, and a code of ethics. These, in turn, are subject to the historical consequences of ideology. Therborn (1980) suggests that ideology only exists in the historical form and that power, ideology, and conflict are always closely connected. Power is hard to capture in any one single definition. As noted by Suominen *et al* (1997), some power is visible and some is invisible, but is closely related to everyday nursing practice. It can be seen as either a relation or capacity; in this case, a capacity to get things done. Both Hewison (1995) and Jacono and Jacono (1994) argue that power does exist within the nurse-patient relationship, but they describe it as being beneficial for care outcomes. This is opposed to the nature of power, which Goffman (1961) describes as suffocating and detrimental to all individuals. Goffman describes power from the point of view of the powerless. It is plausible to think that we exercise power, often usefully (e.g. to separate young people from objectively poor parenting), but then, as the people in power, we would say that wouldn't we?

According to Bowman and Thompson (1995: 228), 'The distinction between management and leadership is important in nursing'. The distinction is often based upon ideological reasoning and cultural assumptions at differing levels. Every nurse will recognise the issue of a top heavy management and insufficient leadership from within the ranks. Bowman and Thompson continue, 'There are too few initiatives for recognising potential leaders and developing them for the future... Following the introduction of the Griffiths Report (Department of Health and Social Security, 1983) and the NHS reforms, medicine has a perception of itself as providing leadership within the NHS' (White, 1993: 228). Is this not the case within child and adolescent provision? Psychiatry and consultant-led services are those which nurses practice. There continues to be a lack of nurses in decision-making positions, and leadership is often equated with ward management or case load initiatives. The criteria for attaining leadership positions remain dependent upon ENB qualifications. The concepts of leadership ability and leadership style have to accommodate these criteria. The traditional functionalist perspectives of trait characteristics and leadership classification, such as, autocratic, democratic, and laissez-faire styles remain valid still as a way of understanding the interactions between leader and subordinate.

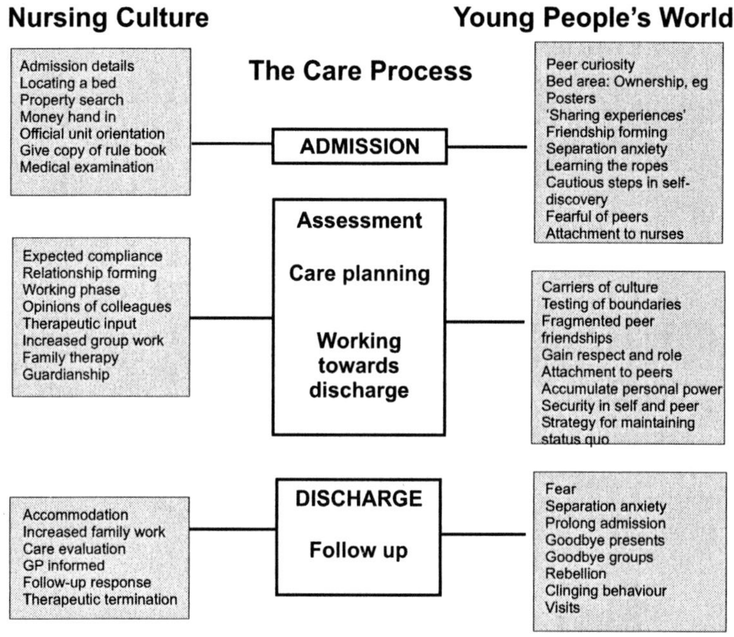

Figure 5.2: Safety in return for liberty

Closing remarks

So you think you're free? Nursing ideology gives us all a sense that we have agency; a freedom to choose; a sense that we have autonomy and the hierarchy within culture identifies the limits or boundaries to that autonomy. Next time you go to work, we suggest you reflect upon the ideological and cultural issues that structure our understanding. Nursing mentally ill young people and children seems, naturally, to provide us with a number of interwoven roles, 'be they shop steward, kindly honorary aunt/uncle, police officer or foreman!' (MP). However, these are not naturally occurring roles, they are manmade. They are constructions with long historical antecedents for both young people and nurses. They appear very natural, but they belong to the twentieth century. Undoubtedly, in the next hundred years alternatives will evolve and carry future patients into the next (M)odernist Utopia.

Chapter 6
The expert, the expander and the educated: advancing modernist concepts

'The literature describing mental nursing in Britain towards the end of the last two decades of the twentieth century employs four terms interchangeably: 'mental nurse', 'psychiatric nurse', nurse therapist' and 'mental health nurse'. The last two reflect an unease with the term 'nurse' which some see as perpetuating the medicalization of those with a mental health problem and the supremacy of the medical model.'

Peter Nolan (1993: 6)

Dialogue

Dean: It seems to be a funny thing.

Sandy: What's that?

Dean: The term advanced nurse practitioner...it seems to say that you have to be something special, better than the rest.

Sandy: What would you want it to be?

Dean: I think it symbolises the icing on the cake. On the one hand it demonstrates nurses' commitment to all the (M)odernist themes of progress, technological advance, identity, and systematic frameworks of practice. On the other, it forgets that these same frameworks are determined by larger structures, such as medicine, psychiatry, power, language, and the fact that good quality care does not necessarily mean advanced care in the scientific sense put forward by modernism.

Sandy: That's all very good, but how will it help nursing ill children?

Thesis for this chapter:

- Individuals are inseparable from the wider world in which they exist
- Nursing assumes the notion of natural selection via the organisation and management of resources. However, a belief in the humanist/Cartesian assumption that effort results in reward masks this discourse
- A dominant discourse in nursing is based upon the construction of a belief in the metaphysical and actual assumptions of order and discipline, as reflected in the needs of the society that is served.

Background and aims

It is hoped that the ideas in this book about modernism and postmodernism are starting to paint a more complex picture. There cannot be a simple account of how being 'cared for' (by nursing science) impacts upon young people, without inclusion of philosophies and theories about nature, society, and the individual. The notion that there is a progressive evolution of progress and truth in what we know is being challenged by postmodernist thought, and nowhere more so than in the priority nursing gives to its elite clinical practitioners, celebrating them in an effort to create a form of high culture; 'high culture' being defined as 'the best' a culture has at any given time during its human history. Confusion regarding what is the best is reflected in the expectations placed upon the boundary-pushing, advanced nurse practitioner (ANP), and the symbolic acceptance nursing gives to the functionalist/manufacturing modern ethos discussed in the previous chapter. The attempt to be modern is a preoccupation more concerned with internal and external power relations rather than with caring for ill young people. This can be seen in the dismissive attitude many working nurses take towards the flag-bearing initiatives of advanced practitioners.

Encapsulated within the notions of 'mental nurse' and 'psychiatric nurse', as noted by Nolan (1993), are other titles that reflect more recent trends. These include: 'nurse therapist', 'nurse counsellor', those providing a description of role, such as 'liaison nurse', 'nurse manager', and those that highlight a particular theoretical approach, such as 'behavioural nurse'. We use these titles to provide us with particular identities and specialisms. These identities separate those nurses working with mentally ill children from those practising with adults, but added to these (as if to demonstrate a reluctance for anything to do with nursing, but everything to do with order, hierarchy, and something which goes beyond conventional nursing) is the title 'advanced nurse practitioner' (ANP). The modernist Utopia is one that inspires this notion of undermining practice, of pushing boundaries, and progressing nursing towards a unified professional paradigm, with its distinguishing titles and distinct roles within the unified profession. The core thesis for this chapter aims to explore the notion that the issue of perceived expert, expanded and educational requirements of child and adolescent mental health nursing form just a small part of the framework that determines the nature of nursing as a whole.

We want to argue that nursing is constructed upon the metaphysical and actual premises of order, discipline, and a belief in the humanist/Cartesian assumption that effort results in reward. In short, the so called work ethic. Such a belief has the disastrous effect of maintaining the *status quo* power relations within the profession, and promoting a pseudo-advancement that may be the only realistic opening available to the expert practitioner. The emphasis must be on this as a reality. This chapter also concludes the large part of our book devoted to ground-breaking. In order to do this it has a number of guiding aims:

1. To explore the current framework for nursing hierarchy and career development;
2. To discuss the issue of specialism, nursing expansion and post graduate qualifications; and
3. To highlight the way nursing has adopted functionalist models of organisation.

Introduction

Child and adolescent mental health nursing finds itself in a similar position to other specialities regarding the issues of career frameworks. Many questions need to be asked and their answers deliberated before the uncertainty nurses encounter with respect to their professional development can be addressed.

Advanced practice, with its determination to spearhead the development of a profession and expand practice into different technological competencies and nursing commodity markets, can be seen as a function of capitalist society generally, as is the pressure experienced by individual practitioners to obtain promotion to higher grades,

- ❑ *What is the current definition of expert practice?*
- ❑ Is nursing a post or a person?
- ❑ What is the difference between expanded and extended practice?
- ❑ Why do we need expansion?
- ❑ How much autonomy do experts have?
- ❑ What qualifications do nurses require?
- ❑ What are the consequences of nursing expertise for other health professionals?
- ❑ What are the future implications for expansion?
- ❑ What part does expansion play in the professionalisation of 'new nursing'?
- ❑ *Is expansion actually reductionist, if it brings specialism in its wake?*

Figure 6.1: Questions, questions, questions.

preferably with imposing titles. The emphasis on growth, progress and meeting wider needs stems from the ritual modern obsession with success, competition for resources, and individual identity. For most nurses, advanced nursing is little more than a buzz word, a fancy idea or the product of bored academics. If this is the case, it is tough and resilient and has continued to grow and overcome all attempts to be ignored. It remains as an icon of modernity, as a process that takes as its standard, 'advancement'. The profession is obsessed with advancement at all costs; however, we urge colleagues to take on board postmodern criticism's questioning not only the models and assumptions that are being advanced, but also the process of advancement itself. Such advancement has not had time to look back and 're-think'. Such is the urgency that the questions, 'What is advanced practice', 'What can it do for my speciality?' are merely answered with the rather predictable slogans of 'pioneering, boundary-pushing practice' (United Kingdom Central Council for Nursing, Midwifery, and Health Visiting, 1993) and 'risk taking' (Patterson and Haddad, 1992). The notions of advancement and expansion appear to be beneficial and realistic goals for future nursing practice in child and adolescent mental health nursing, but they should not be pursued at any cost. It is time to re-think the conceptual issues of what advancement means and what role would nurses need to perform. The usual answer to these questions is subsumed with notions of expert practice, postgraduate qualifications, and increased autonomy. These are the issues to explore because the concept of advancement harmfully reinforces the trends towards hierarchy, power, and fancy ideas for the sake of mere fashion.

Child and adolescent advancement

It is not surprising that nurses working with children and adolescents, in particular, are suspicious of such notions of advancement, because of their historical subservience to psychiatry and general nursing practice. Much of the expansion credited to advanced practice has been seen in general nursing, due to the reduction in junior doctors hours and extra extended duties given to more senior nurses. The idea that advanced practice is about compensating for the absence of medical cover is not what this book perceives as advanced practice. Extension is not the same as expansion and this will be clarified during this chapter. More confusion and disillusionment at practice level appears to stem from uncertainty at a theoretical level. Nursing scholars, trust managers, educationalists, and statutory bodies, including the RCN and UKCC, have always struggled to develop a role and framework that not only advances the career pathway of individual nurses adequately, but separates the distinct specialities of child and adolescent mental health nursing from others, and advances them in a way relevant to their needs. The present model of nurse practitioners (NP), advanced nurse practitioners (ANP), clinical nurse specialists (CNS), and primary nurses (PN) appears to be similar to the model already evolving in the USA. That model extends the provision of practice by taking on medical tasks, yet expands the theoretical knowledge base of interpersonal practice. The model is economical with change to health structures, yet elite enough to require specific graduate and postgraduate education, which allows for selection of candidates by ability. These highly educated practitioners create posts that are evolved according to economic priorities and community needs. However, it is with these central questions that the development of the role currently resides. In order to provide a broad introduction to the nature of these questions, it is important to have some understanding of the way ANP development has been motivated by modernist assumptions, so that we can put ANP in a contemporary framework. We will begin with a brief historical description of the ANP development.

Q: What is the current definition of Advanced Nursing Practice?

A: In brief, a conclusive definition does not exist. What is known is that the theoretical considerations of ANP continue to be a contentious issue at all levels, including academic and at the UKCC. It is, however, perceived that it will be ANP that expands future practice in most specialities; the perverse (M)odernist quest for uniqueness, hence specialities are, paradoxically, related to a false sense of unreproducibility, which modern technocracy aims to mass-produce. Linked to this, a notion of being able to present what is conceivable, but not representable is, according to Lyotard and as noted by Appignanesi and Garratt (1995), the postmodern sublime. The advanced nurse practitioner is the sublime. It attempts to represent boundary-pushing nursing utilising concepts and models that are not in our power to represent. At a practice level, such confusion has trickled down and contaminated the perception of ANP, leaving it struggling to be accepted, perceived as needed, and useful to direct patient care. Therefore, a consensus of opinion regarding its definition highlights the need for ANP to be the 'expander' of nursing theory and the boundary-pusher of practice. The consensus seems to be that the individual ANP, as with other past heroines and heroes, will lead the supposedly necessary advancement, rather than relying on opportunities for progress arising from normal changes in the world of nursing. The modernist cliché depicts specially selected hero-nurses seizing control over nature and make their own destiny. This, however, is a modern dream, because no nurse or other citizen can ever be separated from the wider economic, cultural, and historical conditions in which they find themselves. The advanced practitioner is a manmade notion in the same way that the supposed need to advance nursing within specific discourses is constructed by man. In order to explain our contention in more detail, it is necessary to analyse the work of nursing scholars.

Specialism and the good ship 'Resistance'

There exists within the meta-paradigm of nursing a variety of expanded roles, all claiming to be forms of specialist practice. The impression is that something 'good', progressive or beneficial for the profession is just beginning to set sail from the old world in the direction of the new. This modern age of progress and of the ANP role is accompanied by a feeling of expansion, an expansion that can be likened to those first explorers of the Renaissance sailing west in search of fortune and the mysterious, mythical lands of the Americas. However, the thread that links the various expanded roles and leads them toward a common goal is not clear (Patterson and Haddad, 1992). The following, rather uncertain words written in a paper titled, 'The Advanced Nurse Practitioner: Common Attributes', carry the sentiments of all contemporary definitions of what an advanced nurse practitioner role is, should be, and is likely to be. According to McGee (1993), 'the issue that must give cause for concern is not the lack of novel ideas [from nurses about the possibilities for the ANP], but the lack of clarity with regard to the meaning of these levels of practice in the clinical setting'. Clarification of the situation cannot be sought elsewhere, as noted by the authors (Holyoake, 1995; Holyoake, 1997a; 1997b) and McGee (1993) who said 'it is no use seeking answers in American literature', because it isn't there. The role of the advanced nurse practitioner is new [in the UK] (McGee, 1993), but then the concept is older (UKCC, 1990). It is important to note that very few nursing scholars make reference to the mental health arena. Professor Castledine (1991a) is one of the few and it is with his early support for the role of the ANP in mental health that our analysis begins.

The pond of child and adolescent mental health nursing is shivered by the same tidal wave that roughens the sea of general nursing, the wave being specialism and advancing practice as a nurse-led initiative. The ripples of expanded practice in mental health were noted by Castledine (1991a) who emphasised the mental nurse therapist's role evolving at the Bethlem Royal and Maudsley Hospitals in response to the developments in adult behavioural psychotherapy. He states that 'Community psychiatric nurses also began to develop specialist skills in more diverse ways than the Maudsley model, although general community nurses have tended to view such specialist developments in the nurse's role with great suspicion'. Two years later Castledine (1993) continued to demonstrate his support for ANP by noting that the nurse practitioner had a role with characteristics that often included 'a personal case load, delegated prescribing arrangements, and higher decision-making'. Although he makes no direct reference to mental health nursing, it seems that the call for increased practice autonomy should be universal for nurses. This attempt to provide a 'representational' framework of advanced practice and of how it is perceived is a problem for the nursing scholars wishing to strengthen its acceptability (and uniform nature) by the postmodern. For example, CPN practice is part of an expanded role. It includes taking on facets of medical roles without direct medical supervision. The political importance of such developments at senior nurse level is such that it seems hardly surprising the call for increased practice autonomy and specialism still remains alien and confusing to most mental health nurses.

More recently, the UKCC in its Notification of Practice (1997) was unable to identify a single specialism for mental health. The Notification of Practice has only the heading 'mental health' to cover the whole field of psychiatric nursing .'Proper' nursing, in other words general or adult, has at least 19 categories. It seems that being on part 13 of the register is unlucky because you are doomed to a life long career of non-specialism that may include child and adolescent mental health. You possess restricted skills that occasionally yield a few concepts of bedside manner, which are deemed useful in general nursing. It is no surprise that many child and adolescent mental health nurses gaze towards generalism in hope of finding a brave new world, and see a small island that can be called a specialism in the name of advanced practice. Unfortunately, the sea is stormy and, despite the UKCC, the ship leaks. The sailors are only ever three years from mutiny as they scramble to find five study days. Dependency upon psychiatry and general nursing hinders the self promotion of firmer specialism in mental health nursing. It is a popular comment that 'it's easy for general nurses to be specialists because they have a lot of tasks and things'. It is usually countered with 'we work with people, our skills are people skills'. Whatever the moans and groans, it seems that the main problem mental health nurses have with 'deformation' is a fear of the change and confusion involved in their way forward.

Putting advancement and expansion into a contemporary framework

It seems that the possibilities for advanced nursing practice are real in the nursing care of mentally ill children and adolescents. As with most other specialities, the prospect of increased autonomy, self-management, and supervised implementation of direct patient care is more feasible within the community setting. These are the representations that nurses accept as a workable and progressive addition to nursing duties. Deformation is primarily about abstraction. For example, in art at the turn of the last century, there was great resistance to the non-representational imagery being explored by avant-garde artists. Today, it is accepted. Similarly, the deformation or abstraction of the principal nursing roles within child and adolescent mental health nursing will continue to be aggressively rejected by psychiatry and nurses alike. Hence, at present, the opportunities for expansion of role rather than the concept of expansion at a personal level appears to be the major consideration for creating specific ANP roles. We must clarify what is meant by the titles 'post' and 'role' in order to move the argument for nursing expansion forward. The need to locate some common ground, upon which a contemporary framework of advanced nursing practice in child and adolescent mental health can be considered, is of primary importance if nursing is to be generally regarded as equal within the modernist framework.

At present, most nurses working with mentally ill children are employed by specific health trusts at a particular grade. They belong to a service that is hierarchical, has specific job descriptions, and relies upon a core of skill mix as a foundation for the care provided. Both community and residential care is loosely based upon this model of care provision, which has evolved within all mainstream nursing. Positions are given via interviews, based upon a particular practitioners' experience, qualifications, and the overall needs of the service. Nurses are expected to attain promotion, usually given on the number of years experience they have, educational requirements (and their ability to relate to management), and the possession of certain skills that are usually described as being 'people skills' (as approved by managers). The climb up hierarchical ladders is based upon achieving junior management status evolving into ward management. The individual case loads they carry are fairly divided between team members. Skill mix is usually considered, but the overall model is one that advocates nurses working with a certain number of children/young people at any one time, while managing the unit or assessments, clinics, groups, etc., generally. At present, the scope for expanded practice is rationalised as any activity that is considered special or extra to the norm. For example, the use of more creative work, one-to-one work, active outreach, music therapy, and the use of customised care planning and assessment. This common scenario is, in fact, quite restrictive. Such restriction is the result of a number of complex structures that originate from traditional nursing expectations. For example, as just suggested, the nursing world is not ready for a totalising deformation and deconstruction of its role and theory. It is the view of the authors that ANP is something that, in principle, aims to stretch the traditional norms, but which, in practice, is confined by the same boundaries faced by most nurses. The work ethic of nursing has us assuming that if we work hard we can advance ourselves beyond expected limits, do more for the our young people, gain respect, demonstrate autonomy and freewill by breaking the boundaries that have always de-professionalised nursing in the eyes of medicine and the public. However, postmodern criticism, rightly understood, gives us a truer picture of our working lives, even as it increases our ontological insecurity.

Individual role not post

The ideology of (M)odernist advancement emphasises that ANP can only be fully achieved if every individual practitioner recognises his/her personal responsibilities, firstly, to him/herself and then to his/her patients. ANP is about roles; that is, personal roles in providing the basic art of nursing and expanding the knowledge base of nursing in child and adolescent theory. These personal roles consist of the things nurses do every day that benefit their patients, and the dissemination of ideas. The ideal practitioner would have the aim of finding out more and making personal management strategies that attack the complacency of assumed practice. This is the widely understood, yet false assumption of (M)odernist progress. It is a myth because, as with the 'death of the author', modern child and adolescent mental health nursing practice (with its emphasis on specific key service roles) just legitimises and re-confirms the power relations between people and the broader discourses of psychiatry. The postmodern paradox is, however, that roles, although commonly viewed as being specific to individuals, are similar to posts and titles (which are largely camouflage and sweeteners to individual nurses to take an active role in maintaining existing power relations). The ideological pressures take the form of statements about moral judgements. It is often argued that what really counts is the personal attributes each nurse brings to the child, regardless of his/her grade, post or role. When highlighted in such an altruistic way, it would be very hard for most nurses to disagree. But this argument is not as plain as it appears. It has, beneath its surface, a philosophical foundation that is in line with the overall philosophy of this entire book.

We claim, centrally, that the individual can and should overcome and transcend the power-relationships that are otherwise inseparable from interaction in society, including (of course) the interactions between nurse and patient. The individual is a whole, with the ethical responsibility to think and act with the benefit of fellow man in mind, embodies the notions discussed in the earlier chapter about humanist/holist principles that belong to a philosophical tradition of the constructivist/constructionist paradigm, and which has been openly accepted within nursing. Accepted uncritically! Therefore, it comes as no surprise that any advanced practice will be seen as the responsibility of individual practitioners. But how can individual nurses be responsible for the decisions made by chief nurses sitting around board tables, pondering issues that appear to be so detached from actual practice? Expanding individual practice is one thing, expansion of a profession, another. Too much excitement becomes tied to the idea that nursing can express itself with the aura of the ANP post, a high profile specialist practitioner, worthy of admiration and serious consideration; that then becomes more important than the care role. The totalising effects of ANP development have overshadowed the expressive roles that nursing pioneers intended. Fully realised, the ANP conception minimalises expressive roles to the point where they are eliminated. This ambition of 'reformulating' nursing is, and will continue to be, inadequate to represent a nursing reality. It is unrepresentable; a sublime reality or hyper reality that offers us a picture of mass (re)produced, ready-made, advanced practitioners, displacing the very idea of the originality and sacred uniqueness so important in nursing epistemology. The idea of installations and 'the power of display' has become far more important for nursing, hence the ANP's difficulty in actually achieving recognition. The failed attempts of deformation have created reproducibility associated with the mass production of the modern. The idea that the modern can only exist as a reflection of the postmodern (the so called Postmodern Condition, Lyotard (1984)), therefore, reflects the way nursing attempted to make the concept of ANP by deformation a reality. ANP has succeeded in producing a mass (re-produced) non-original icon of (M)odernist advancement, with the idea of ANP being more important than the reality. The process of this development can be highlighted in the merits of how nursing leaders continue to sublime concepts within the modern framework of technology and progression.

Expansion and extension

In 1993, at the Heathrow debate, a group of chief nursing officers and nurse leaders considered 'The Challenges for Nursing and Midwifery in the 21st Century' (Department of Health, 1994) the 'new modern era'. Eight strategic issues for nursing and midwifery were identified to highlight how nurses might be affected:

- What will be the context in which nurses work
- What will be the contribution of nursing to meeting the needs of individuals
- How will substitution impact on the role of nursing
- How will the public react to the changed role of nursing
- How will teamwork be developed with other carers in the health and social care spheres
- How will professional accountability, authority and responsibility be altered
- How will regulation impact on quality
- What will be the implications for initial education and training, retraining and continuous training?

As noted by Schober (1995), a key word is 'substitution'. In the pursuit of effectiveness and efficiency, the report stated that substitution relates to the location of care and tasks. The report recognised that the reallocation of tasks between nurses and other professionals is almost inevitable. This reminds us that nursing is generally considered within a multi-disciplinary team (MDT) model. The specific management of such a team (it should be noted) is almost always consultant-led, thus highlighting the power differentials between the professionals within the team. It is usual that roles and responsibilities for care delivery to the child or young person are decided by the medical profession, regardless of the hopes and expectations of those who truly believe MDTs create a forum for a blurring of roles, a type of fuzzy inter-disciplinary team. It has to be said that nursing is secondary to psychiatry, even if the consultant does seem to listen and often publishes work referring to the special qualities 'his or her' nurses possess. The frustration of working in such a hierarchical order is reflected in the nature of the safe task and taxonomic rituals in which nurses are involved. Every young person will know what a nurse does and does not do. Therefore, the expansion vs extension debate has to include consideration of such task allotment.

The Scope of Professional Practice (UKCC, 1992) is of significance for nurses, because it states that, any 'enlargement or adjustment of the scope of personal professional practice must be achieved without the compromising or fragmenting of existing aspects of professional practice and care' (Section A 9.4). Therefore, any pushing of boundaries and expansion of practice must be 'additional' or must 'complement' that which already exists within the scope of nursing. The issue of role extension (e.g. taking on medical tasks) brings with it the pre-conditions of skilled practice and attendance on courses as one would expect, but this serves only to extend practice rather than expand, enrich, or deepen it. Properly understood, expansion is far more complex and intricate than learning the task of taking blood or prescribing paracetamol. It revolves around the understanding of those philosophical as well as theoretical concepts of nursing, which ultimately make sense of our practice. These concepts include: issues of nursing diagnosis, the art of nursing and evaluation of actual practice, and nurse-led research. What the Scope of Professional Practice permits is the opportunity for all nurses (including those in child and adolescent psychiatric nursing) to critically analyse practice and strive for full potential at both a personal and professional level. However, it is precisely that 'Scope' which infringes upon the individual and advanced practice. For the modern has brought to nursing issues of safeguards, social agreements, and the protection of all from all. In an effort to improve standards of care, attention has turned to the standards of post-registration education.

The expanded role

It is consistently assumed that, where advanced levels of nursing skill are developed, they are associated with beneficial outcomes. This post PREP period is a vacuum in child and adolescent mental health nursing. Service development post-HAS (1995) has not been sufficiently established, so the case for the ANP role has not been tested or recognised within a changing culture. Both expansion and extension are a process of change from two conceptual standpoints. For the purpose of this discussion, the definitions of both are taken from the older work of Murphy (1970). Role extension is defined as a unilateral lengthening process, role expansion as a spreading out or a process of diffusion. Both change processes are evolutionary in nature, in that the body of knowledge and the field of practice are constantly emerging. Moreover, both change processes are directed toward the same goal: meeting more adequately the health care needs of our society. The unilateral extension of the nurse's role to incorporate delegated functions might appear to be one answer to the shortage of medics, but for nursing it holds long range implications—in our opinion, mostly negative—in that nurses will continue to be the handmaidens of medicine. On the other hand, role expansion, taken literally, implies multi-directional change. Expansion as a process of role change is undertaken not only to fill perceived gaps in the health care system, but also to promote new and pioneering components or systems of health care (Holyoake, 1998a;1998b). This brings up the question, 'Why do we need advanced practitioners when we've never had them before?' The answer still remains uncertain even after 15 years of debate in the UK. It could be argued that most nurses are unaware that ANP is now considered a third level of practice in the same way as clinical nurse specialism (CNS) and primary practice (UKCC, 1994). This lack of understanding reflects the continuing ambiguous nature of the role; to us, the role cannot be filled in one way for all specialisms. An example of the tedious nature of the past 15 years of development is highlighted by the fact that, until recently, ANP was considered the third level of practice; however, the authors argue that there cannot be a universal model of ANP, but rather one that is specific to the micro-paradigm of a given specialism, such as child and adolescent mental health. This fragments the current guiding theory that ANP can be standardised and monitored (on North American lines) and promotes, instead, the guiding philosophy of individualism. Hence, advancing practice can be seen as far more important than being an advanced nurse practitioner.

Criteria for ANP: Advancement and the ENB Course 603

For nurses in child and adolescent mental health services, there seems to be a small, but significant amount of nurse development that is educational-led. This is the traditional ENB Course 603 Child and Adolescent Psychiatric Nursing. Criticism of the ENB 603 has been made by Symington (1997: 9) who states 'the ENB 603 course no longer prepares nurses to look after and treat disturbed children and adolescents'. Such an accusation is worthy of point, but seems to offer no solution to improve the undefined preparation he thinks necessary. He continues, 'I am not convinced that it enhances the practical skills of nurses' and adds 'Nurses need to develop and extend their knowledge and skills in this speciality'. A number of points

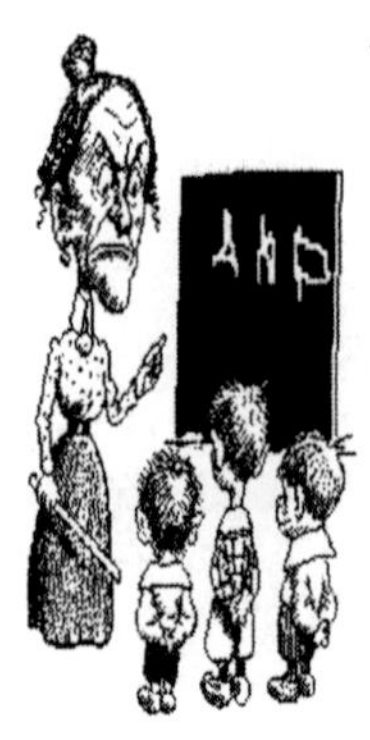

regarding the ENB 603 should be discussed in view of the concerns expressed by a number of nurses (not necessarily Symington, who highlights the debate), who view the academic pioneers of this now more demanding course as Zealots. The first being that all criticisms are made without any relevant alternative being given. It is not good enough to exclaim that nurses need to extend their knowledge and skills. This is not a solution, it is a concern. It is also interesting that the concept of extension is used rather than that of expansion. Secondly, it is no secret that the ENB 603 course continues to be and has always been the golden ticket to promotion. The difference is that now the course requires a higher and more significant level of reflection and academic understanding. How can this be a bad thing? Would the critics have us believe that the ENB 603 should teach practice-based tasks to nurses who should not question why they are doing what they do? That would be an absurd waste of time. Advancement is not just about being a good nurse, it's about doing well informed nursing and knowing one's capabilities. Critics would have us all believe that the ENB 603 is irrelevant because it doesn't 'teach the right stuff'. In fact, what is really being quibbled over is the fact that most ENB 603 courses now offer academic qualifications, such as a degree or diploma, which the old ENB 603 (Pre 1991) didn't. Managers no longer control the academic input into the speciality and this is an issue for the whole service. Likewise, the students have no choice about the nature of the course—they can only hope and 'plot', as noted by Pursey, that it will be them who get picked to go on it next. Thus, the relationship between practice and educational content that has guided child and adolescent nursing still belongs firmly in a domain that is far from settled, and continues to be disrupted by issues of power discourse.

Child and adolescent nursing has progressed a long way in the last twenty years, regardless of the theory practice gap that many critics of the ENB 603 would have us recognise, but its identity still belongs firmly within the paradigm of general mental health nursing. This, in the general public's view, is also secondary to general nursing. It shares a broad epistemology about human behaviour, care needs, and nursing interventions derived from the generalist education nurses' experience. Nurses working with adolescents will talk about 'utilising Peplau' in the same way adult nurses do. Therefore, although, as we have seen, advances have been made, it seems that the time is ripe for nurses to consider the nature of their role in the spheres of both practice and theory.

To do this we have to ask some secondary questions; these include: What makes a child and adolescent mental health nurse different from any other mental health nurse; What makes a child mental health nurse different from one who works entirely with adolescents; What is ANP in child and adolescent nursing; How is it different to other roles?

- ❑ What makes a child and adolescent mental health nurse different from any other mental health nurse?
- ❑ What makes a child mental health nurse different from one who works entirely with adolescents (Think CPN)?
- ❑ What is ANP in child and adolescent nursing?
- ❑ How is it different to other roles ?

Figure 6.2 : What makes a child and adolescent nurse different?

Facets and qualifications of child and adolescent advanced nursing

At present in child and adolescent mental health practice, the ANP role remains wide open to interpretation and can be moulded to fit specific needs; this is, in itself, ambiguous adding to the resistance and apparent apathy encountered when new clinical roles have been introduced in the past. Therefore, the primary aim of any child and adolescent ANP is to promote acceptance for the role. Such a task may not be feasible without managerial support. Every nurse would expect a charge nurse to be an expert in his/her field regardless of whether or not he/she had an ENB certificate to prove it. They would expect a ward manager to have years of experience and know what to do in a 'crisis' and to have more ward-based autonomy than a staff nurse. Even a first year student nurse at the bottom of this safe hierarchy has clear expectations regarding role, but ask any mental health nurse what the ANP role is and confusion will be part of the response, followed by a sigh of 'oh, not another type of nurse'. This brings to mind the clarification of role described by Andrews (1989) as 'equal but different'. The task of the ANP role in theory is concerned with pushing the boundaries of the pond, but in practice the advanced nurse practitioner may find it easier to convince nurses that sharks don't bite. This is synonymous to the pre-revolutionary stage in which nursing, as a paradigm, finds itself in comparison to medicine. It may well be the case that mental health nursing cannot ever belong to the same paradigm as general nursing, and its specialisms cannot be regarded or viewed in the same framework.

Q: *What qualifications will the ANP require?*

A: It is important to acknowledge that distinct 'areas' for specialist and advanced practice 'not levels' of nursing are given by the UKCC (1994). Such areas are hard to distinguish from one another, but involve a minimum first degree level and continued clinical input, preferably a practitioner attaining Master's level qualifications or above. Armed with these criteria, with their map, and a compass, mental health nurses can set sail in search of new worlds.

The adventures mental health nurses face include the attainment of a first degree and, as ambiguous as it seems, the role is presented as being detached from hierarchy, as though it is an individual endeavour when mental health ANPs struggle to implement direct clinical practice. The facets of supervision, assessment and diagnosis of particular patients on a referral basis, teaching sessions, and the management of research projects are just a few that mental health nurses would recognise as they brave the elements, but, in order to succeed, they would have to overcome the weight of tradition. Inevitably, tradition will test them and tempt them to succumb with the 'so what?' question. Tradition says that these supposedly new skills are being performed by the charge nurse/sister now. In what way would the ANP role push more boundaries? Tradition casts doubt on the difference between a role and a post? And surely expert practice should be striven-for in preference to any degree, even if those degrees introduce the dawn of 'new nursing' and the all-graduate profession?

The 1960s saw the rise in scientific and medical knowledge, advances in technology, and the advent of para-medical specialities, and also influenced professionalisation. The adoption of delegated medical tasks by nurses may have been an attempt to assert a higher clinical status and the RCN (1988) pioneered the concept of the extended clinical role of the nurse. However, this was never meant to involve losing sight of the commitment to the art of nursing care, but it appeared to encourage the rise in 'technical' commitment rather than the intended specialist knowledge under the auspices of the CNS. The 'domain of nursing knowledge' is a range of interrelated components that are essentially theoretical and practical. The central phenomenon of the nursing domain is the interaction between nurses and patients and how nurses respond to individual and group needs. The interaction between patients and their environments consists of nursing activities and competencies that focus on the health and nursing needs of patients and their families. This scientific interpretation does not take into account the three other types of knowing offered by Carper (1978). These are aesthetics (the art of nursing), personal knowledge, and ethical knowledge.

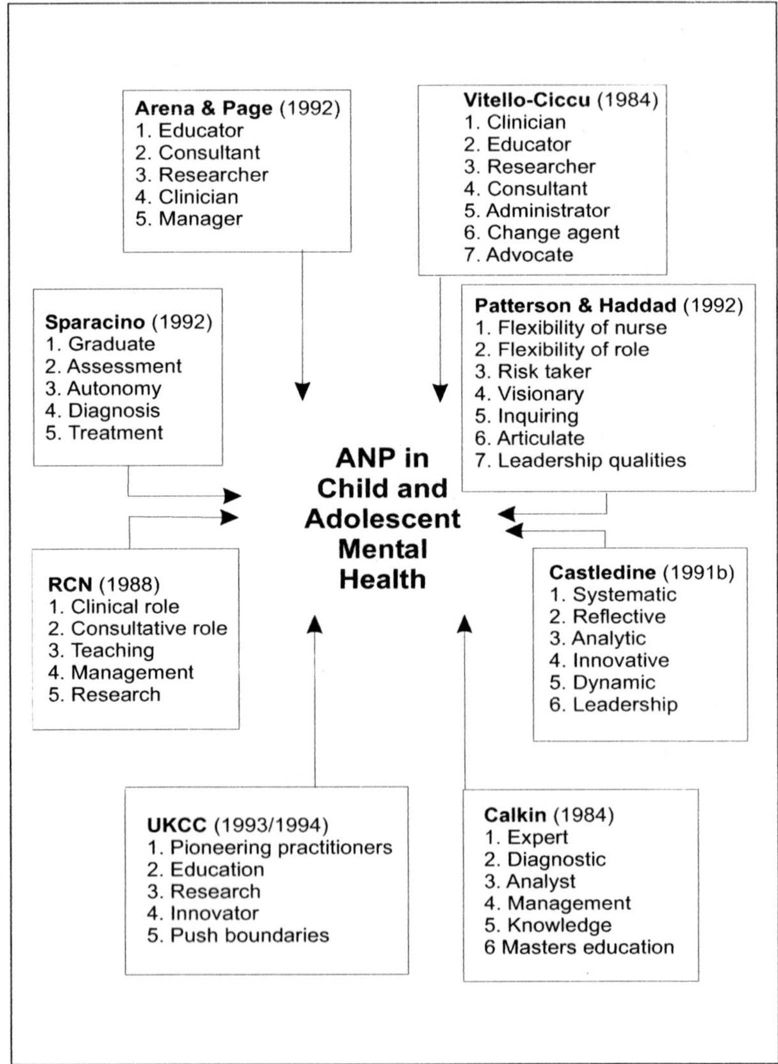

Figure 6.3: Facets of the ANP role—the mass (re)produced aura of the role

Q: *What are the core facets of ANP?*

A. Can we formulate general principles to tell us which facets of ANP are useful and which are not? Discussions of this question are less fruitful when carried on in isolation from other related questions. Are there any general principles to tell us when a nurse becomes an ANP? Nurses will say it is when they are expert or when they have completed the necessary ENB course and fulfilled the requirements of the UKCC benchmark, but the two do not necessarily relate. Why is there thought to be a difference between one being an expert practitioner, but another needing MSc academic qualifications to prove it and, on top of all, a post which specifies a Masters as job requirement. If the new nursing profession needs specific practitioners to be innovative and boundary-pushing, whose duty is it to ensure that such concepts become a reality? Clearly, at present it is the academic and statutory councils (UKCC, ENB, RCN) who are deliberating over an American model of ANP. Management and trusts are encouraged by the supposed economic advantages of providing a routinised framework, but is this the correct model? It is one that will, inevitably, involve the two main debates of extended vs expanded role and post or person. How high a priority should this be given?

Many people think that a discussion of this kind, arguing about the merits of specific practice levels, is either superfluous or else impossible to resolve. This is often because they make one of two false assumptions: the first is that there is one set of 'true' nursing beliefs, which no informed nurse could reject once understood. This view makes all discussion redundant. The other assumption is that theoretical arguments and the practice of nursing are so subjective that no useful discussion can take place between those who differ.

Who is the expert practitioner?

It is widely accepted that, within trust structures, 'it is not uncommon for managers to be appointed from among the senior clinical staff who carry managerial and supervisory responsibilities in their professional, clinical practice' (HAS, 1995: 129).We assume that the ANP role comprises a number of facets. These facets belong to primary areas of practice, but may overlap with specialist areas of practice. Most child mental health nurses practise with high specifications of skill, so what determines the assumption that they may not qualify for the ANP role? It seems that the determining factor is education at first degree level. However, in practice and according to Sparacino, (1992), 'to acknowledge that there are no gradations between the novice and the expert, some practice settings have instituted clinical ladders, a promotional system which uses both objective criteria and a peer review process to recognise and reward excellent and advanced nursing practice'. To become an expert, you must accede to and internalise the mental health nursing culture, find your role models and 'learn the ropes'. More often than not, the ritual is laid down by your 'expert' colleagues. It is by their say-so that you 'join the exclusive club' and achieve expertness. This is an issue discussed in the Heathrow Debate document (Department of Health, 1994) and the advent of ENB measurability in the form of courses has superimposed a higher value-system upon this highly questionable popular culture. Some suspect that educationalists have been creating experts like monarchs creating brand-new aristocrats; all-too-often we hear the remark: 'she's brilliant at the exams, but can't nurse for toffee', thus highlighting the theory-practice gap. As a way forward, we want to argue that psychiatric nursing is a highly diffuse and difficult activity in which many earnest nurses engage with great seriousness. It is not a concept for picking out any specific activity (as hinted at in *Figure 6.1*), but for laying down criteria to which a family of activities must conform in both theory and practice. The central questions worthy of note are: 'How do we identify an expert nurse in the first place' and 'Do all and only those who are identified as experts make use of intuitive judgement in the way that Benner (1984) describes?' These questions dictate the specific competencies for the

(1) Perceived expert practitioner *within a speciality with a* post registration training *at* degree level
(2) Continued clinical practice *within at least one* specialist area
(3) Developing economically viable liaison networks *within the* wider care trade
(4) Leading consultation role
(5) Advancing pioneering nursing diagnostic procedures *within a* speciality
(6) Develop relevant teaching *within specialities*
(7) Initiate and co-ordinate nurse-led research
(8) Management

Figure 6.4: The official (M)odern criteria for advancement

psychiatric ANP role. Below is the representational mode for recognising the modern ANP.

Core skills	Specialist	Advanced
Honesty	Accepts emotional risk	Development of policy
Active listening	Focussed knowledge	Enforcement of policy
Problem solving	Accepts uncertainty	Evaluation of policy
Relationship skills	Questions theory	Nursing diagnosis
Care co-ordination	Undertakes research	Boundary definition
Use of protocol/framework	Expert in a specialism	Research co-ordination
Acceptance of support	Supports change	Initiates and leads change
Advanced empathy	Influences policy	Research dissemination
Assists research	Junior/senior management	Specific knowledge
Team working	Awareness of ambiguity	Supervision and liaison
Care planning		Leadership and support
		Philosophical
		Autonomous

Figure 6.5: The tri-archy of nursing for mental health nurses

These lists can not be considered definitive and represent the simple ideas of the authors. What they are is a measured attempt to provide a framework to help nurses categorise practice. The issues of expertness, management, teaching, and research are the broad considerations.

Conclusion

This chapter has attempted to widen the debate in advanced practice and put forward a position with respect to mental health nursing. The emphasis has been upon the importance of the psychiatric culture, which has always limited the autonomy and perceptions of individual practitioners. It has also (we hope) emphasised the ambiguity of the legitimate development of the role and, thus, highlighted the need for mental health nurses to take the initiative and seize the opportunity to forge their own role. Ideally, that role would not attempt to dress the old up as new, but incorporate core facets relevant in practice. This debate will continue to expand as the role does, but hopefully, as a result of positive reports, rather than from the 'one down position' in which this chapter suggests mental health nursing finds itself. The notion of the ANP as the cutting edge of nursing development has to be considered against the fact that it has eliminated all elements of expression. It is possible that ANP was conceptually postmodern before it became (M)odernist dogma. Now it has become a type of conceptual icon contaminated by elitism and energetically marketed, mass-produced, and represented as a 'new nursing'. Against this, we put the cry from the majority that it isn't nursing, but rather the experimentation and creation of a perceived modernist need. In postmodernist terms, ANP is just another movement towards nursing's self-annihilation. ANP has attempted to move beyond the representation of nursing into what cannot be represented; ANP imposes duties perceived not to belong to nursing, and beyond the ideas of dreamers: nursing as a medical equal in the eyes of the general public. When nurses call for 'back to basics', they not unnaturally show dissatisfaction with the experimental and chaotic—if only because these are not being well enough sold, or marketed in an attractive enough package.

Chapter 7
The evolution of attachment: the nature of power

'...industrial capitalist societies have evolved complementary ideologies of attachment, which have stereotyped...relationships in remarkably gender - differentiated, and spatially segregated categories"

(Marris 1991:185)

Dialogue

Dean: What do we know about attachment theory?

Sandy: Well, we know it has been important for the practice of child and adolescent mental health nursing for over 30 years.

Dean: Doesn't it argue that there is a biological basis for the attachments of infants and children with their mothers? There is certainly research that demonstrates this.

Sandy: All these aspects are important, but it is also important to recognise that its development coincides with the development of interactional and relationship theories of the humanist school.

Dean: We need to consider this and the links made with attachment theory and child and adolescent mental health nursing.

Sandy: It won't be possible to analyse the effects of attachment in one chapter though.

Dean: I know, but it is possible to highlight some of the issues associated with it and consider the postmodernist debate.

Thesis for this chapter

- ❑ Attachment theory belongs to a (M)odernist project

Background and aims:

The theory of attachment, principally developed by Bowlby (1969), has within it an evolutionary status, notions of power relationships, and a historical development in relation to the theories of behaviorism and functionalism of the mid twentieth century. These three concepts are of central concern to this chapter and will be discussed in relation to the postmodernist perspective. It is argued that postmodernism illuminates neglected philosophical structures relevant to the application of attachment theory in practice. As such, this chapter pays attention to the uncomfortable aspects of attachment as opposed to its usual connotations of usefulness. To do this, it will first consider the evolutionary and historical developments of the theory followed by a discussion of its constraints. The two aims of this chapter are:

1. Trace the links of attachment theory to its foundations in romanticism and psychoanalytic theory; and
2. Explore the philosophical and evolutionary status of attachment theory.

Principal assumptions of attachment theory

Attachment theory stresses the responsiveness of the child to its mother; this is said to be internalised by the growing child. It is assumed that the child begins to build up an idea of the self through this process and is, therefore, understood to have a naturalistic and instinctual epistemology. In the modern sense, attachment theory has been emphasised as the brainchild of Bowlby (1969). Its central tenet presupposes that a distressed individual will naturally seek security and, in mental health, it has been stated by Holmes (1993) that the very fact someone seeks psychotherapeutic help implies they will have had difficulties in establishing such security in the past. Within child and adolescent mental health services, nurses are the largest group of professionals working in this area and, in residential centres, it is they who spend most of the time with these young people (Barker 1974). It is widely seen that nurses are placed in a particularly valuable position to offer nurture to some young people who have, perhaps, not received it in the past. This can be demonstrated by the philosophy of nursing care, which has been identified by the staff at the Lowit Unit in Aberdeen, who perceptively express the need for specialist nurses to become involved with attachment issues. They state:

> '...*The aim of the nursing staff is to help children develop and explore different strategies to deal with their difficulties, which allow the child to develop their potential as human beings. This is hopefully facilitated by providing a warm, nurturing environment, where the child is accepted as an individual with individual needs. The opportunity is provided for all children*

> *to develop and maintain a meaningful relationship with a member of the nursing staff of their choice. Through this relationship the individual child can be helped to develop a sense of 'self worth' ...'*
>
> (Paice, 1996: 63)

Central to this self-worth is the attachment process. This philosophy embraces Bowlby's views of attachment, but also includes the additions made by Winnicott (1990), who perceived the way to self-worth and responsibility for others as a developmental progression. This progression commences in the infant's experience of a caring environment and the ability of the mother to 'hold' the environment. Winnicott included the whole perspective of protection, caring and containing that embraces emotional and physical survival. Then attachment patterns can be seen to emerge from the dependability and responsiveness of this holding environment.

Fahlberg (1981) suggested that setting the pattern for attachment behaviour begins at the prenatal period. This is when the parents begin to develop images of what the child may be like. Factors, such as the pregnancy (both timing and quality) and the relationship between the parents, together with their own experiences of attachment and parenting, can affect this process. Once the child is born, the attachment process continues through the interactions between mother and child. The attachment behaviour is organised around the need to maintain proximity to the attachment figure. Once there is a threat, attachment theory presupposes that a distressed individual will naturally seek security. Proximity-promoting behaviours have been identified as sucking, smiling, clinging, visual attention, and crying upon separation and, as such, proves to promote positive contact (Erwin, 1997) Thus, the attachment figure will hope to provide a secure base from which the child can explore the environment and to which he/she can return at times of stress and discomfort.

The child's attachment behaviours are based upon a schematic cognitive representation of the child and carer relationship and is identified as the 'internal working model' of attachment. This internal working model influences the way the infant perceives and appraises attachment-related information and affects the ability of the individual to plan future action. The infant goes on to develop expectations about his/herself and about others through the use of these working models. The self is accordingly viewed as either worthy or unworthy of care and protection, and caregivers are viewed as available to provide care and attention (Bowlby, 1973; 1980). Bowlby proposed that attachment begins to evolve into goal-corrected partnerships. In these, the child is expected to balance and integrate flexibility in his/her own attachment needs to the caregiver. The child moves further away in order to explore his/her environment and then starts the complex process of relying on mental representations of attachment rather than the actual presence of the attachment figures. Finally, the goal-corrected relationship that emerges during the preschool years can set the scene for attachment across the life span (Crittenden and Ainsworth, 1989). As the child grows toward the teenage years and adulthood, the internal working models of attachment are expected to reflect an increasing understanding of the caregiver's own motivations, feelings, plans, and developmental goals, and this should result in a relationship of mutual trust and understanding. The principles throughout the attachment process rest in safety first and exploration later.

Observations of the child's response to separation have been used to describe ways in which individuals cope with threats to their environments. Many researchers draw our attention to the studies completed by the Robertsons (1952), whereby separation from the attachment figure has evoked greater proximity-seeking behaviour. Children being placed in strange environments with experience of prolonged separations from their attachment figures have been shown to demonstrate a series of transitional behaviours. First, there is searching and calling for the parent and, after a while, children become quite desperate and show what has been interpreted as a state of mourning. Once the caregiver returns the child has been noted to turn away and appear uninterested, holding fast to his/her proximity-seeking behaviour. When the dyad is reunited this disattachment is often reversed. The child may shortly after become clingy or demanding and afraid to let the attached figure out of his/her sight. As reassurance is given, the more securely attached behaviour is reinstated and the child is then free to explore autonomously. Thus, it depends upon the caregiver's responses to the uninterested behaviour and/or the clinging behaviour. Clearly, the child's behaviour can be very distressing for the caregiver, but if this uninterested behaviour is mirrored by the caregiver towards the child, then a return to a reciprocal secure relationship is difficult.

Investigations into these patterns of attachment have been undertaken by Ainsworth (1967; 1978) both in Uganda and in the USA.

These experiments were set up in laboratory conditions within a playroom, and observations were made of brief separations of mothers and their children who were at the time aged approximately 12 months old. This test, designed to evoke attachment behaviour, is known as the Strange Situation Test. The mother and child were requested to play together in the playroom with a researcher present. Following 20 minutes duration of playful interaction between mother and child, the mother was requested to leave the playroom for a few minutes, while the infant stayed in the room with the researcher. Upon the mother's return the reunion takes place and then both the mother and the researcher leave the room for another few minutes before once again returning to the child. The whole situation was video taped.

Power and constraint

So, attachment is a function of the infant-parent relationship, but can also be suggested to reflect the emotional security craved for as a product of the twentieth century. In particular, it may be bound up in Euro-American notions of individual needs and interpersonal relations. It has been suggested that the categories of attachment behaviour identified in Ainsworth's Strange Situation procedure might present the moral judgements of a particular society at a particular moment in time, rather than generalising to all humans throughout time. (Harwood *et al*, 1995). Correspondingly, Grossman and Grossman (1990) began to question this reliance when they replicated the Strange Situation test in Germany, and concluded that a large portion of 'normal' infants were classified as 'insecurely' attached. In addition, social class studies have demonstrated differences in attachment behaviour. Ogbu (1981), for example, observed that parents from low socio-economic situations offered warmth and affection towards their infants, yet used a severe and inconsistent style of parenting with physical punishment. The middle-class parents were observed to offer a softer style of parenting, which incorporated a style of explanation and negotiation of rules. The researcher suggested that this is a reflection of the different social expectations of distinct environments

Philosophical and evolutionary status

As noted in parts of the book so far, postmodernist critique emphasises the evolutionary status of modernism, particularly psychological and sociological frameworks of understanding. This is, in part, due to the belief that man cannot be separated from his wider culture and history. The work of the attachment theorists utilised the epistemologies and methodologies of the natural sciences. Thus, the theory of attachment is, today, based upon notions of what it is to be natural in a modern society. It forms one strand in a twentieth century tradition of exploring supposedly instinctual concepts of what it is to be human (in particular, a mother). As noted by Smith (1997), Lorenz's work on aggression, together with a cluster of other empirical studies by authors, such as Ardrey and Morris, emphasise the desire to find a basis for human action beyond politics and the socialisation of modernity. That search continues to hold strong appeal, a type of quest for an inherited animal nature. This is not in itself a bad thing, because attachment theory has enabled and initiated a revolution in how we, as nurses, view the therapeutic relationships we have with children and young people. Although this is not contested, the evolutionary nature of modern psychology and how we view our world, together with the social relationships in it, has enabled an over-enthusiastic and speculative reliance on it. This can be seen in its synthesis with models of human relations in nursing. The developments of natural science helped set a precedent for the way interactions and attachments are viewed. The insistence on quantifying, providing frameworks, and gleaning more information from natural sources, which could be transferred to the benefit of mankind, emphasises attachment theory's historical development within the philosophical framework of functionalism. When reinforced by biological determinism, it can become an excuse, as Smith (1997) says, to 'legitimate political inequality and social injustice'. When Bowlby presented his theories of attachment, he was part of the advancement of studies in ethnology, whereby he drew parallels between apes and human behaviour. The general feeling was one that acknowledged the importance of the instinctual drives, already described by the psychoanalytical sections of the psychological paradigm during the turn of the century. The aim of ultimately discovering some clues to the evolutionary nature of cultural society via the study of instincts provided yet another technology, or gateway to the proof that science and progress were near to understanding the nature of man. The relevance of this for child care has been apparent since attachment theory's widespread adoption. Nurses, today, view it as one of the most fundamental tools available to them in practice, because it justifies the therapeutic relationship and the strong attachments they make with the children and young people they care for.

As previously discussed, functionalism has a premise that man, society, and scientific knowledge can mirror the natural structures and functions of nature. Hence, the perceived similarity between attachment theory and the work conducted by biological anthropologists. The determinist nature of attachment theory reflects functionalism's want of observable and useful pragmatic solutions to man's relationship with fellow man and society generally. The horrific effects of the Great War (1914–1918), and the subsequent political revolutions that followed, provoked a feeling that man had been stripped back to his animal instincts. The increased interest in the dark and mysterious inner-world was nothing new, as Freud and the Vienna Circle attempted to provide a scientific basis for understanding the nature of man. A pessimistic view of that nature seemed to be supported by the growing socio-political unrest during the first half of the century. As a movement, psychoanalysis and the culture of the twentieth century allowed a dynamism, which Marxist analysts (Frankfurt School), particularly Marcuse and Adorno, saw as a means to link material conditions, social structure, and the individual's psychological identity to what was thought to be the most natural thing of all: instinct. During the early days of psychoanalytical development, a distinct but sustained theory of child developments was proposed by Klein. This contributed towards a separation between the notions of adulthood and childhood and the increased sense of developmental issues, generally. Klein's work stimulated research on how babies in the first weeks and months established relations between their needs and the object: the mother. Thus, a growing emphasis upon the bond between child and mother was encouraged. The support for Klein from the Tavistock Clinic, in particular Bowlby's insistence upon the importance of the mother- child attachment, reveals the legacy of such modernist thought today. In their attempt to provide a well rounded and scientific framework, the object relations theorists led to a mainstream theory of personality which, according to Smith (1997), encouraged a 'post-war political hope that welfare provision would achieve a civilised society'. Hence, the socio-historical conditions encouraged the dissemination, the reception, and the interpretation of attachment theory, which, in turn, led to the social aspects of attachment being interpreted as being in the realm of the mother/infant dyad. Construction of the 'natural' also constructs what is unnatural if taken for granted, and the enlarged responsibilities placed on mothers tend to neglect the wider social perspectives. This neglect actually reduces the choices under offer and can lead to stigmatisation of the mothers who fail to measure up to ideal domestic expectations.

Conclusion

This chapter has had the aim of identifying the philosophical and evolutionary roots of attachment theory. We hope that we have provided the means to encourage dialogue and discussion with respect to the important developments and assumptions derived from attachment theory over time. In conclusion, the reader may be left thinking that the biological determinism bound up in our twentieth century notions of instinctual drives comprises at least some part of the way we care for children and young people; that is, there is some foundation in the idea that we are biologically driven. This is a universal belief that seems to fit with what we have all observed and which many have reported in nurses' experiences during their work in the clinical area.

The method for discovering 'scientific truths' about human nature has placed the theories of development and attachment firmly within the empirical and positivist paradigm of enquiry. As Foucault (1967) emphasised, stating a truth is not just an occasion for transmitting information, but also contains and exercises power.

The biological and mechanistic notions of human life, coupled with the claims made by functionalism and behaviourism to have a modern Utopian insight into the care and welfare of children and young people, only emphasise the conflict within psychology and the demands made of it by the public's expectations. The evolutionary theories of human nature, together with the powerful assumptions arising from them, have been more than just tolerated; in some areas they have been accepted wholeheartedly, in order to prove that a hierarchy of social relations may be fully justified by 'science'.

Deconstructing social arrangements can help to draw attention to a variety of aspects not included in empirical studies, aspects that may be hidden (for example, power relations.) The constructions are, therefore, allowed to be viewed as meaningful narratives rather than psychic reality, thus authorising attachment to be redefined as a capacity to form and maintain relationships and trust throughout our lives, but to be seen as a capacity that is not fixed or unchangeable.

Section III: Critiquing modernist concepts: A postmodernist project

Aims for this section:

(1) To argue that real mental illness is just a product of psychiatric diagnosis. Nursing has for a long time argued that labels do not give a valid or 'truthful' representation of reality. They are symbols of power and authority and are best studied by critiquing the metaphysical assumptions placed upon them; and

(2) Psychiatry as a discourse is best considered a form of social control with ethical pretensions ('moral medicine and gate keeper of society').

Chapter 8
The ~~Schizo~~, the ~~Starver~~ and the ~~Slasher~~: deconstructing the labels of psychiatric metaphysics

"...the practice of 'subjectification'; the subject of the text or category actively participates in a discourse that constrains and regulates their lived reality."
Parker *et al* (1995: 91)

Dialogue

Sandy: We've talked a lot about the nature of postmodernism, but we haven't talked about deconstruction or discourses in their historical sense.

Dean: No, but the obvious way forward is to highlight the contribution of deconstruction as a method of critiquing language, metaphysical concepts, and the judgements made by health care professionals in everyday practice.

Sandy: We need to give a historical description and also talk about methodological reductionism.

When John (aged 15 years) was admitted to the adolescent unit for assessment, he didn't have a medical diagnosis. As such, there was nothing wrong with him but, with stubborn persistence, the care team were certain they could find something suitable. He needed to be assessed in order to receive his label, to qualify him for his sick role, and to be deprived correctly of his liberty. The way his body was perceived and examined at this micro level is instrumental to how knowledge is constituted regarding his label. His parents were more than happy to allow the 'specialists' to help him control his anti-social outbursts that disrupted their home life.

When Jane (aged 14 years) was being treated for anorexia during a seven month admission, she was subjected to an environment which kept her out of sight. It offered the hope of holistic nursing care, yet only gave her the behavioural rewards she earned.

When James (aged 15 years) was discharged from the adolescent unit, he'd spent a total of two months under close surveillance for his self harming behaviours. He had been empowered by the powerful to choose to be a participating individual in the same society which had contributed to his deviance. His sense of his own existence was distorted by uncertainty about the boundaries of his mind, and those of his body; he was tormented by dualism.

This chapter will examine the concepts behind the care received by John, Jane, and James during their stay in residential care. The central thesis is that the dominant philosophical discourses of methodological reductionism and holism (phenomenology) are founded upon conflicting assumptions, which have consequences to how mental health and illness is perceived.

Thesis for this chapter

- Individuals are viewed as quantifiable single units of analysis, e.g. the notion of specific characterisation of psychiatric diagnosis, such as schizophrenia. However, individuals are inseparable from the wider world in which they exist
- The main philosophical ideas that dominate psychiatric nursing are holism (phenomenology) and methodological reductionism; however, these are founded on conflicting assumptions that have harmful consequences for how mental health and mental illness are perceived.

Background and aims

The aim of this chapter is to explore how caring practices maintain a balance between long-standing opposing tensions; i.e., how caring professionals assume that whatever they do is ultimately beneficial for their patients because it appears logical, rational and, therefore, legitimate. This chapter, like all the others, does not attempt to locate 'truth'. Rather, it uses techniques, suggested by deconstruction, to unravel the contradictions between the metaphysical assumption and practice that exist in the care of children and young people. It aims to use basic deconstructive principles drawn from the work of Derrida (1976) and Foucault (1971; 1980), in particular, the philosophical concern with labelling and defining health. The deconstruction of these two concepts enables a better understanding of the issues thrown up by the care offered to John, Jane, and James. Each of these young people experienced the full force of modern day institutional Tier 4 care. This brings them in touch with issues relating to their freedom and to being labelled and then classified as mad. This chapter has three aims:

1. To provide a brief discussion regarding the nature of deconstruction as a particular Postmodernist method for illuminating metaphysical inconsistencies between method- ological reductionism and holistic practice;
2. To argue that the symptomology experienced by John, Jane, and James amounts, at best, to no more than a poor excuse for allowing psychiatry to exert social control and, at worst, will reveal that the professionals involved, woefully, lack theoretical understanding of what they are doing; and
3. To argue that classification of symptomology maintains the metaphysical assumptions upon which they are founded, only at the cost of suppressing valuable, if differing points of view— hence, at the cost of patient well being. The public gets what the public believes it needs.

The development of deconstruction

In order to progress further, it is necessary to define how the term 'deconstruction' is used in this chapter and how it can be used to analyse the mental health care provision offered to the three young people. This is not a straightforward task; as noted by Collins and Mayblin (1996: 4), the answer to, 'What is deconstruction?' is difficult to find because there have been many misrepresentations of its use and definition. Some of these have varied from the simple comments, such as, 'it's a way of doing philosophy' and 'a way of reading theoretical texts', to rejections of its ability to do either, 'its the latest fashion in literary theory' and 'it's a positive device for making trouble'. Therefore, although many scholars of philosophy have commented upon deconstruction in its relatively short life, since the mid 1970s, the only thing they agree upon is that its originator is Derrida (1973; 1976; 1982; 1988). (It is also necessary to acknowledged the important contribution of the post structuralist, Michel Foucault (1971; 1975; 1977; 1978; 1980), with his discourse analysis, as noted by Parker *et al*, (1995) and Henderson, (1994)). As French academics, Jacques Derrida (b1930) and Michel Foucault (b.1926; d.1984) were very much part of the modernist and post-modernist fever in French universities, but what Derrida offered was not just more post-modernism, even though he is usually credited with being one of the school (Lechte, 1994: 105). (In fact, as noted by Collins and Mayblin (1996: 16), his writing 'has no extractable concepts or method' unlike Foucault. Hence, its lack of definition and consensus of opinion regarding what deconstruction has to offer). Therefore, this chapter uses the term 'deconstruction' in a similar way to Parker *et al*

(1995) and assumes that its driving priority is to identify the fault-lines in the metaphysical assumptions behind labelling and defining health (central to methodological reductionism) of the three young people. However, it should be borne in mind that deconstruction is more than just a close examination of poor practice.

Derrida (1973) spoke of deconstruction using the foundations of a house as the actual weapons to destroy it in the absence of anything else. Bearing this in mind, his work follows two strong threads of thought, which we can also apply to a critique of modern psychiatry. First, *derailed communication* and, second, *undecidability*. These two threads are of direct relevance to the premise of this chapter, which is that the care offered to John, Jane, and James is dominated by methodological reductionism (positivism) and holist philosophy as a result of conditioned and naturally accepted assumptions about the world (see *Figure 8.1* for a historical account). It is the metaphysical assumptions of these two philosophical traditions, as with all western philosophy, that Derrida aimed to disrupt at their foundations and by doing so dislodge the certitudes and 'turn aside its quest for an undivided point of origin' (Collins and Mayblin, 1996: 47). Derrida never said that the task of disproving metaphysics was possible or even relevant, but he acknowledged that metaphysics pervades western thought (Wood, 1992). These assumptions include the universalities sought by positivism and the quest for complete systems in holist philosophy. As such, metaphysics suddenly becomes very relevant to the care of John, Jane, and James, and the thousands of others being cared for in psychiatry. But how is it possible to begin to shake the foundations of mainstream thought in psychiatry and western philosophy?

According to Osborne and Edney (1992; 178), one way is Derrida's move to blow up structuralism's pretensions to have answered all existing questions. These answers involve the structures within historical discourses that can be located primarily in language and its uses in culture. For Derrida, these hidden structures are only metaphysical constructs and their exposure utilises a framework similar to methodological reductionism. It is important to note at this stage that Derrida criticised Foucault's (1973) work on madness by questioning how someone could defend the right of the mad to be mad, while using the concepts of the oppressor. Even so, Foucault has proved to be one of the most important figures in critiquing the discourses of psychiatry, although not credited (or discredited) as being a deconstructionist. In a similar vein, Derrida viewed the structuralist rival phenomenology with as much suspicion. Its belief in the inner structures of consciousness, as proposed by Husserl (1982), as a means of revisiting central ontological questions (Heidegger, 1958; 1962), and the development of existential philosophy from these tenets (Sartre, 1992), all have one thing in common with respect to metaphysical propositions. According to Derrida (1967), the whole edifice of existence or presence relies on the metaphysical opposition of 'inside/outside'. This is a universal structure, therefore, a human construct that neglects certain oppositions in favour of others, and the holism underlying the treatment offered to John, Jane, and James belongs to a tradition, which, like methodological reductionism, is based upon a metaphysical tradition that their ~~'illness'~~ is within, possibly caused from without, but needing recovery at the hands of experts. Related to this foundationalism are the unresolvable differences between phenomenology and structuralism, which centre upon two primary considerations. First, their differing conceptions of meaning (Collins and Mayblin, 1996: 58) and, second, their different projects. Phenomenology posits meaning as an interior consciousness, whereas for structuralism it arises in the relations between units of language. With regard to their larger projects, phenomenology is a philosophy of the internal consciousness, whereas structuralism is a relational theory of language and culture (Collins and Mayblin, 1996: 58). Derrida's aim was never to try and resolve these differences, but rather to expose the difficulties of neat *dichotomies* and *foundationalism.*

The method of exposing these dichotomies and shaky foundationalism utilises the method of deconstruction, that is, using the foundations as weapons. As a method of analysis, deconstructionism has been put forward in many guises. These include 'moderate' and 'radical' versions (Fuchs and Ward, 1994) to 'exposing contradictions' in and implications of theories (Parker *et al*, 1995: 131). This assignment presents a version similar to the moderate. It unravels some of the explicit assumptions within discourses, in particular, methodological reductionism and holistic practice. Therefore, as noted by Wheeler (1995: 181), the definition of deconstruction that we use is, in effect, a demonstration of the incompleteness or incoherence of a philosophical position; that is, the positions of methodological reductionism and holistic practice. This definition reminds us of the sentiments of Derrida who acknowledged that moderate deconstruction is not deconstruction, because it embodies foundationalism (the posit of first principles or assumptions) (Agger, 1994; Norris, 1987).

Methodological reductionism	Holism
Methodological reductionism is one consequence of a science based upon close observation and experimentation. Although the conditions of scientific methodology are not our concern, it is important to note that, as a philosophical tradition, modern health care has a two thousand year history. For example, the Greek philosopher Hippocrates (c450–c370 BC) and his colleagues may reasonably be classified as scientists, for they believed in close empirical study of health and illness, similar to medicine and nursing today. However, this classical Greek medical view of health and illness was primarily holistic as opposed to reductionist. It was the era of what can be termed the sickman. Medicine was focussed on the whole human being. There was held to be just one cause of all morbid phenomena. This classical medical monism came in two forms: humoral theory and solidism. The human body was thought to be in a state of equilibrium, a view that persisted until the nineteenth century. The idea of a body of trained professionals sharing collectively in the best scientific knowledge of their day and drawing on the medical authority from their membership of this group or 'college' took root in Italy in the late fifteenth century. However, scientific medicine still had very few cures, but it was gradually developing a rigorous methodology as it discovered new classifications of disease. The history of medicine is the history of distinguishing one condition from another. Over the past two centuries, definitions of diseases have shifted from the nature of the symptoms and signs, to the underlying changes in the tissue—the pathology—and from there to the chemistry of cells and tissues. Treatment, however, was not forthcoming during the rise of industrialisation; so bleak was the outlook that therapeutic nihilism flourished. To the therapeutic nihilists,nature itself was the best cure, there was no need to intervene for most illness was self limiting. In short, the development of antiseptic consciousness and magic pharmaceutical bullets, the development of psychological theories by Freud, Klien and the domination of psychiatrists in psychotherapy , as noted by Rowe (1990: 11) made sure that the sickman had begum to disappear	As noted by Kolcaba (1997), 'The holistic health movement encompasses divergent philosophies, religious doctrines and psychological theories. It is so diverse that practically every theorist can claim holistic credentials'. As already noted, the idea of holisms is not new. The Greek scientists and mediaeval thinking thrived upon humoral holisms. In the fourth century BC, Plato (1968) and Aristotle (1966) articulated versions of this doctrine (Kolcaba, 1997). However, the growth in methodological reductionism to produce certàinty resulted in the decline of holistic theory. Today, nursing has a determination to view every patient as a whole. This is linked to the metaphysical holist notion that reality is comprised of wholes. Nursing argues that care should take into account the subjective experience of the individual as well as the social, biological and medical considerations. The suggestion is that medicine is over concerned with biological considerations at the expense of other important considerations. As such, the philosophy of holistic practice is not anti-medical, rather anti-reductionist, usually at the level of interpersonal considerations. As noted by Wynne *et al* (1997), 'One factor that may have contributed to the present state of affairs concerns the epistemological approach adopted by nursing.' Traditional scientific empiricism has been the epistemological basis through which almost all knowledge of the natural sciences has been derived. Other approaches to knowledge development that are more accordant with the holistic philosophy belong to the sociological and behavioural sciences (Kramer, 1990 cited in Wynne *et al*). This highlights the intention of nursing to focus on caring rather than cure. The underpinning concept of holism is the acceptance that health is determined and defined by inter-related social, psychological, and biological factors (Wynne *et al*, 1997)

Figure 8.1: Historical development of methodological reductionism and holism

Foundationalism

What is foundationalism? Foundationalism in the philosophical sense holds the view that knowledge and epistemic justification are two tiered (Moser, 1995: 276). In brief, this amounts to knowledge being either inferred (as with phenomenology) or deduced (as with positivism). The popular beliefs in this age of science are based upon two metaphysical premises. These are the binary oppositions of presence/absence and origin/supplement. For Derrida, experience itself is a combination of a presence and absence. For example, non-being is experienced as part of being and is not to be found in the Platonic essence, which would be revealed by a special kind of philosophical quest (Palmer, 1997: 134), one that aims to discover an unchanging origin. For example, James received care, which argued that he had suffered trauma early in his short life. Therefore, by seeking the origin and exorcising it, a new sense of being would occur. These holistic pretensions are wrapped up in cause and effect notions, which continue to dominate psychotherapeutic metaphysics, metaphysics that utilises a language of oppositions and relations to argue that James needs psychiatric treatment. This is typical of logocentric prejudice. As noted by Collins and Mayblin, (1996: 47) regarding such metaphysics, Derrida recognised that he had some allies, notably Heidegger (1962), Strauss (1978) and Freud (1997), but he asserted their reliance on metaphysical assumptions, such as unconsciousness and its opposite consciousness, and the logocentric prejudice in theory. He makes specific reference to both Strauss (1964) and Saussure's (1994) demonstration of logocentric prejudice (the privileging of spoken sound over script) (Derrida, 1976; Johnson, 1997: 32).

Science, medicine, and psychiatry all share this assumption that the discovery of knowledge needs to be logical (Holyoake, 1997b; 1998c; 1999). From all directions, from cereal packets, magazines and daytime television, the images about health that assault our eyes and ears repeat and repeat again: health is the same as fitness. It is on this logical level that Derrida attacks metaphysical assumptions of the written and spoken concepts, which rely upon signs, repeatability, and relationalism for their usefulness. That usefulness is already part of the metaphysics of presence and origins. As such, no one can ever escape from logocentrism, but, as noted by Palmer (1997: 133), 'we can at least reveal what is, in fact, obscured and repressed by that metaphysics'. We can recognise a metaphysical system similar to structuralism's binary structures, which privilege one of the two poles of these necessary binary opposites. James is deviant because he cuts as a symbol of his distress. If we say 'distress on the inside leaks out', we make a metaphysical assumption.Universal dreams about health, such as a belief in a Utopian or ideal state of health, can all be deconstructed in relation to their absent opposites (which are stated as being not healthy, or dangerous to health) In addition, the authors would argue that the political sensitivities of psychiatry and medicine are phenomena that often go unrecognised. All three of the young people were removed from society in what was deemed to be an appropriate attempt to protect them and society. However, as noted by Coleman (1998), 'Psychiatry has rooted itself in a tradition based on, at best, pseudo-science… it is not based on what can be called natural science'. The borderline between therapy and social control is a fine one. As an opening of argument, this now requires further analysis and deconstruction.

Social control

> "But I don't need to be HERE !" He turned his attention back to the locked door and began repeatedly kicking it. His face was flushed red and tear stained.
>
> "Don't be silly John. You know that you've got to be here because the doctors think things are wrong." The nurse sighed as she spoke and looked over her shoulder at her colleagues who were hovering just in case John needed restraining.
>
> "What the hell do you know, you're only a nurse."
>
> "I know that this type of behaviour means you'll be here longer."

Deconstruction tries to show that, in all cases, the prioritising of one set of beliefs over another displays mere cultural manipulations of power, and to show that, under deconstructive scrutiny, these oppositions break down and collapse into each other (Palmer, 1997: 134). John's anger and confusion stemmed from the fact that he had been abandoned by his parents in a strange place. He had no freedom and he had no label. The fact that he didn't really want a label of schizophrenia did not halt the process of assigning him one. That process is at the core of methodological reductionism. The medical model is committed to the concept of individual diseases, which medicine defines by identifying collections of signs and symptoms. For psychiatry and its growth from medicine, this symbolism, which in John's case was the hearing of internal dialogue and aggressiveness, led to Foucault's 'Ship of Fools' (1973) eventually coming into dock because, as noted by Palmer (1997: 101), the ship is 'no longer a ship but a hospital'. The classical age was changed to a logical one by psychiatry and with it the classification of symptomology. As a discourse, society feared those like John, Jane, and James because they were no longer romantic fools, but rather a symbol of 'anti-nature'. The cure being work and strict moral order and reason, which psychiatry attributed as treatment. John, therefore, bore a two hundred year history of treatment, which has only been cushioned a little in our time by the introduction of watered-down holism and child-centred care. The main structural machinery of language and culture handed madness over to psychiatry, but, despite this silencing of the mad, society fears the label 'schizophrenia' because it is one of unreason. Today, that unreason is often seen as being pre-determined by the patient's genes. For John, as opposed to Jane and James, does not have a choice if he is tormented by voices, whereas the latter are viewed as having a choice, to eat, or to stop cutting. This behaviour is often thought to be the natural punishment of a moral evil (Foucault, 1973). This emphasises the complex web that the marvel of psychiatry has spun for itself; for what it has achieved is to encroach upon normal human conditions. Normal conditions require language to organise them, but, as noted by Palmer (1997: 112), one of the main themes of Foucault's work begins to unfold: the threat of unreason and the notion that madness is always a threat to (M)odernity (madness is an historical artefact). The use of labels enables society via the policing of psychiatry to organise, protect, and defend against the un-preventable modern threat of madness. To do this, the mad man has to acknowledge that he is mad and hold himself responsible for being so.

This raises two points for Derrida; firstly, Derrida (1976) attacked the whole 'nature' versus 'culture' distinction in the west because it is already 'part of the metaphysics of presence and origins' (Palmer, 1997: 132). Nature, and therefore madness, is just part of a hierarchical semiological system of signs. John, Jane, and James are seen as children who need to learn respect for patriarchal authority. The work ethic and family ethic will be reconstituted in the asylum. The power of medicine is in the clinical gaze; that is, the body is an object of inquiry and the individual is a case (Henderson, 1994). Power is maintained through the surveillance of activities; normalising judgement is the practice whereby individuals are required to conform. Secondly, Derrida (1974) examined the limits of language'. By doing so he searches for the author in the text and concludes that interpretations are based upon metaphysical foundations. The medic's hand-written assessment forms for

John, Jane, and James incorporate these interpretations. All three require their label due to the threat (the modern threat) they pose to themselves and society, in the same way he bestows his expertise. As noted by Erwin (1997: 60), the growing scepticism about discovering objective epistemological standards is in response 'to the perceived failures of logical empiricism'. Expertise in John's case is related not to the presence/absence of illness, but to the 'scientific' standing of the illness, to being able to demonstrate the illness's very existence (see *Figure 8.2*). This leads us to a second theme: the presence/absence of John's, Jane's and James' illness.

Concepts of health and illness (Aim 2)

> "When I cut myself I sort of feel ...er..., sort of free. You know, in control and relieved." James was sitting in the clinic while a nurse applied a dressing to his fresh cuts.
>
> "I don't know if I want to understand why you do it James... What I do know is that there are other ways to help yourself." The severity in her voice slipped out and cut deeper than a blade. She had intended to be sympathetic and non-judgmental...perhaps even supportive towards the whole situation James found himself in.

The study of the classification of disease (which is under constant revision) is nosology, and underlying the question of nosology is the question of ontology, that is, the existence of things in the real world. Today, the major ontological battle is over the status of mental disorder—does it exist at all? If so, can different types of disorder be classified in the same way as physical disease? This discussion of the ontological status of diseases flows into a second problem area. Where does a disease originate? Medicine and psychology have tried to understand the confusion related to the biological and to the 'mind'. The roots of this body/mind dichotomy run deep in modern western philosophy. These difficulties of nosology and ontology, of biology and mind are reflected in the problems of diagnosis. We are reminded of Foucault's (1973) premise of being, which reiterates our great fear of 'modern madness'. When Jane's mother tearfully asked if her daughter was mad, all she had to do was look at the hospital environment, the seclusion of her daughter, and the doctor's stethoscope. These are the signs confirming madness, which metaphysically remind us of the tenuous link between the body and the mind. One sudden movement can dislodge the unity, creating madness. It is only psychiatry that can put us back together again and keep the madness away. The analysis of social control and power relations continues to repeat itself at a functional (see

Goffman, 1961; Parsons, 1951), political (Coleman, 1998) and post-structural level (Foucault, 1973), highlighting the metaphysical foundations that need illuminating. Sociological writers attempting to explain these differences, according to Parker *et al* (1995: 40), 'tend to resort to a fundamental dualism linked to the fact that society is discriminatory'. This highlights the metaphysical notion of individuality vs society, and the absurdity of attempting to undermine theory using similar theory that is interwoven into the same foundations. It is similar to building bigger and more rickety houses on the same foundations rather than living with the anguish of philosophical uncertainty in the 'house that Jacques deconstructed'.

How one defines illness is part of one's belief system and is largely determined by one's culture. When James cuts himself, his behaviour cannot, we maintain, be classified as a disease. Diseases are abnormalities in the structure and function of body organs and systems and thus are a problem of biological malfunctioning. Illness, on the other hand, is perhaps used as a better description, but has to be considered with caution. When James describes his feeling of release and control when he cuts, it conjures up concepts of illness because he describes these subjective experiences that are open to expert interpretation. He is seen as sick because his behaviour is perceived and experienced by the social group as being abnormal or even deviant. Whether James considers himself well or ill is a matter for experts to deliberate, regardless of his personal ontological experiences. His symptoms are easily detected as being deviant to the norm, and so seem to require his legitimised loss of freedom and personal choice. It is likely that such behaviour in medieval Europe would have been described as a result of witchcraft and as having a supernatural cause. Today, he is diagnosed as having depression with aggravated personality difficulties. This type of logical ordering is what Parker *et al* (1995: 37) have described as 'enshrining abnormality'. The underlying argument is that, in order to relieve suffering, there is a need to be able to do something about it. This focussing on the form rather than the content makes James 'workable' and 'practicable'. It objectifies, making it present (presence/absence) and giving it a cause (origin).

La differance: Locating the opposite (Aim 3)

> "Go on, just try and make me eat it. I'll throw it all over you".
>
> "Don't talk to me like that young lady. You have to eat in order to live".

The discourse (discourses can be seen as sets of statements that construct objects and an array of subject positions, Parker et al (1995). Discourses always entail relations of power).

	The Labels *John*	**The Labels** *Jane*	**The Labels** *James*
The Labels	Psychosis Aggressiveness Delusions Inability to Interact	Anorexia nervosa Sexual abuse Obsessive compulsiveness Irrational fear of weight gain Extreme academic pressure Rigid family dynamics Control issues	Suicidal/depressed Developmental issues Attachment issues Poor social ability Low self esteem Low frustration tolerance Physical/sexual abuse Neglect Poor economical status High intelligence Chaotic family dynamics
The Process	Increased observations Medication Assess risk Reduced freedom	Weight gain program Limits on exercising Medical monitoring Abuse of privacy Close surveillance Forced feeding	Special observations (Restricted privacy) Restricted freedom Alienation Medication Peer isolation Limited school
The Assumptions	Danger to self Danger to others Anti-biological/anti-nature	Danger to self Inside out (letting out the emotion Dysfunctional learning Success is felt as failure	Danger to self Danger to others Limited coping strategies Re-learning Inside out
The Hidden Assumptions	Freedom No other services Medicine is full of experts It's better than a police cell Chemicals as a cause Compliance-refusal to conform (Marxist) Its not your fault Don't listen to the voices	Family handing over responsibility, e.g., fear of death itself Help me make sense of all this mess Surveillance (the gaze) Science rules, OK	Self destruction is wrong The State takes privilege for destruction Encroachment into normal human response

Figure 8.2 : The House that Jacques Built

The foundations of the argument for Jane involved the metaphysical sentiments that nourishment is good and the ontological question of 'to be or not to be'. It is better to exist than not to, and besides you don't have any choice because 'you're mad'. These are the concepts typical of those to which Derrida would apply la *differance* (notice the spelling with an 'a' which Derrida provides on purpose in order to distinguish it); that is, a tactic to disrupt the daily routines of language and meaning. It represents undecidability. Using this tactic allows for analysis to question the metaphysical assumptions behind the analysed. The reader should have noticed that some written words or signs have been crossed out throughout this chapter. This has not been a mistake. On the contrary, it has been quite deliberate. Putting words under erasure (borrowed from ~~Heidegger~~) allows it to be both there and not there, cancelled, but not rejected, present and absent. Given different circumstances and another historical period, the diagnosis of all three young people would be different. The use of erasure allows nothing to be ignored, dismissed as non truth, because there is no such thing. For John, Jane and James, truth is different, and for those caring for them. Which is right—the methodological reductionism and its label, or the subjective experiences of the three young people? What deconstruction and erasure allows is the identification of these confusing phenomena all the way back to their metaphysical foundations. Therefore, both culture and Jane's ~~illness~~ can be treated as real things. Jane must be observed by the psychiatric gaze and display appropriate cultural attributes to the norm. For example, she must keep herself safe by eating and then engage in the talking cures to get her 'inside' out. As noted by Hepworth (1994: 181; taken from Parker *et al* 1995: 48), 'the gendered nature of anorexia and bulimia nervosa is thus regarded as incidental rather than essential and fundamental'.

Conclusion

Putting the question, 'What has deconstruction got to offer?' under erasure demonstrates the uncertainty of its practical application for John, Jane, and James. They all find themselves in an uncompromising position. They exist within the psychiatric machine; a part of the state that, if deconstructed metaphysically, is not based upon the logic claimed for it. If we re-visit *Figure 8.2*, it is possible to note that the assumptions and the hidden assumptions are those which can be deconstructed. What this chapter has highlighted is that John, Jane, and James's presentation can be viewed as (1) derailed communication, and (2) undecidability. These are the two major themes of Derrida's deconstructionism. They are also to be found in the realms of methodological reductionism and holist philosophy. This leads us to consider the metaphysical foundations of 'the assumptions' (see *Figure 8.2*). The belief that both Jane and James' illness can be relieved by bringing the inside out and the idea that John's ~~schizophrenia~~ is anti-natural emphasises the two themes of this assignment: (1) labelling, and (2) social control. This chapter concludes that both have metaphysical foundations rooted in mainstream positivism and holistic practice. As authors, we diametrically oppose the usual 'reality' in which medicine (and nursing) offer solutions built upon these foundations. Instead, this chapter offers an alternative or an opposite introduction, one that, if taken to its extreme, would argue that mental illness does not exist, but is relative. At its most practical, however, it encourages practitioners to examine the broader discourses (see *Figure 8.2*) at work in psychiatry and then focus on the small changes in practice. For example, we could acknowledge the pernicious results of the Diagnostic and Statistical Manual of Mental Disorders's (DSM) and the World Health Organisation's International Classification of Diseases' (ICD) attempt to categorise human experience for the sake of conceptual tidiness. Although Derrida emphasises the need to use the component bricks as weapons, such a feat is seemingly impossible and unrealistic with a sky scraper as big as psychiatry. But even as we haunt its long corridors, we can ask why we need to have the doors labelled 'Schizo', 'Starver', and 'Slasher'; perhaps we can replace them with John, Jane, and James. This postmodernist concern with a return to individuality and representation has not been fully explored within this book, but a brief introduction to the ideas about foundationalism, la differance and their use in practice via the discourse fulfils some of our aims. Deconstruction is not destruction, rather it is the first stage of a more and better considered construction.

The notions of foundationalessness, constructivism and La Diffarence, by themselves, produce a negative epistemology, that is, they tend to make us doubt what we think we know, or dissolve knowledge altogether. They do, however, emphasise in their critique of the norms governing the care of John, Jane, and James that all knowledge should be considered as equal—apart from political power (Lyotard, 1984)—and this highlights the commanding position that psychiatry has cantilevered out for itself from the firmer structures of medicine. The labels and the subsequent treatment afforded to John, Jane, and James do not adequately represent the neopragmatist post-modern conclusion affirmed by Lyotard or other post-modern thinkers. Young patients, like John, Jane, and James, do make choices, can lead lives and be happy in a 'knowing how to' way rather than a 'knowing what' way, these being usually thought of as biological, social, and psychological laws (whether universal or not) that affect them.

Chapter 9
Introducing Mr Authority, Mrs Containment, and Little Miss Individual

'If you want to get ahead, You've got to get a hat'.

Maggie McDonald CNS (1997, Personal Correspondence)

Dialogue

Sandy: When we think about authority, it's usually about being in charge or being able to get others to do a task. It's the legitimacy of a rank or role.

Dean: Children do as they're told because that's what they're supposed to do...'seen and not heard' and all that stuff.

Sandy: Yes, but there's also a belief in the West—which youngsters share—that young people and children have legal rights and equality, and certain freedom. The question is 'how much power do they have?'

Dean: Most freedom comes in the form of being allowed to 'get away with things'. Most exhibited authority seems to be based on a commonsense model. So this chapter will look at the interpersonal level, and how power is thought to be a commodity that effects us all, especially children and young people.

Sandy: Yes, professional power similar to the 'expertness' we've examined.

Dean: It is assumed that, in this modern age, authority is a two-edged sword. On the one hand it shouldn't be used to the detriment of individuality, yet, on the other, it is seen as a last resort or down played as a means to a utilitarian end. We celebrate individual rights, yet impose air bombardments in the Gulf, all in one fell swoop.

Thesis for this chapter

- Psychiatry utilises authority to re-normalise rather than treat. It is a socially constructed discourse that is more about power relations than the relief of mental illness
- Nurses utilise the power they inherit from their privileged position to reinforce moral judgements reflected by society at large
- The nature of individuality, when examined at the point of conflict with society, highlights the issue of authority in nursing.

Background and aims

This chapter examines one of the fundamental issues related to contemporary child care and the care provision for the mental health of children and young people; that is, the concept of authority. It will be argued that authority is a complex and fundamental entity, relevant for consideration in its own right. We believe it is central to the dominant discourse of psychiatry, which regulates the interaction between individuals, be they young patients or nurses. It is proposed that personal authority for both children and nurses can be viewed as internal and intra-personal constructs of everyday life. As such, it embraces having the authority to make decisions, make changes, take responsibility, and take mastery for the future. In nursing, authority is thought of as a kind of moral commodity; for example, getting others to behave in certain required ways by appealing to rank, seniority, or experience. These serve to improve an authoritarian view of what the current social necessity might be, and also license subsequent warnings and threats of 'terrors o' the earth' if there are signs of non-compliance. In practice, this is often reflected in the way behavioural models utilise the basic instruments of reward and punishment, as seen in the plethora of literature related to good behaviour and behaviour management issues.

Aims

1. Debate the issues (philosophical) of individualism in relation to authority; and
2. Explore how the concepts of power and authority are made available to nursing personnel by psychiatric discourse.

Introduction: individuality, authority, and autonomy

The exploration of individual authority in terms of the interpersonal transactions between nurse and child or young person is poorly researched (with the exception of attachment or developmental research). The assumption is that nurses exercise authority within a trusting relationship in order to contain, teach, and direct behaviour, so that the child learns to respect and comply to the rules of society at large. All this is presumed to be beneficial for social interaction and for allowing the child to survive and have his/her needs met. The underlying assumption is that youngsters would not be in contact with Tier 4 services if their social needs had been met and they had learned social compliance.

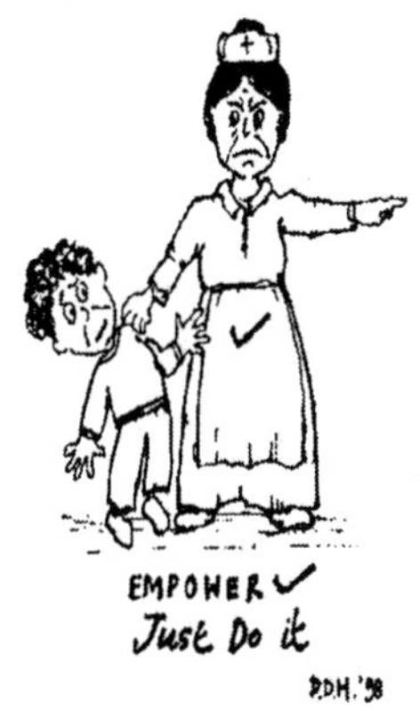

In an attempt to analyse what the concepts of authority and autonomy mean in practice, it is necessary to break down the related issues to provide a starting point for a postmodern critique. The issue of individuality provides us with such a point, which can be seen to be at the very foundation of what it is to have authority and autonomy. A study of the individual, be he/she a nurse, young person or everyday citizen, is at the core of the authority debate and is formulated upon the central questions: 'What is the relationship between the individual and society' and 'What does it mean to have authority?' These questions need to be put, although they can never be fully or conclusively answered. They encompass many of the empirical and metaphysical philosophical issues that have been debated for centuries, but are still central to direct individualised caring, to modern practice, and to the way care provision is organised as a whole. As noted by Kvale (1990: 42), modern thought concerns the 'quest for external legitimation, the dichotomy of the universal and the individual, the opposing of a technical rationality to a romanticist emotionalism, and the issue of quantitative commensurability *vs* qualitative uniqueness'. Take the example of nurses using philosophical approaches, such as phenomenology, existentialism, and hermeneutics, to understanding the situation of a child who is admitted to a Tier 4 institution, and who may be encouraged to take an active part in his/her own care and be autonomous. Aaccording to Kvale (1990: 42), the misuses of such philosophy will 'often come to serve as external sources of legitimation rather than as radical new ways of conceiving of the human subject and its relation to the world'. Opportunities to correct the balance between the individual and the 'institutionalised community' would then be missed. Therefore, in order to consider interpersonal authority and autonomy in depth, it is sensible to tease out the core philosophical issues to form part of a postmodernist critique. The two core issues are first, individualism as the basic prerequisite of living a (M)odern life, and second, the postmodern rejection of originality. This unfamiliar notion is, in fact, an important element of our political, legal, educational, and health care institutions. It is the interplay between individualism and the use of power by nurses as a fundamental facet of caring for individuals that this chapter now examines.

Individualism

To begin establishing if to be an individual incorporates issues of either authority and autonomy (or a combination of both), it is necessary to show that individuality is an existing reality. A general contemporary assumption is that each individual is significant, can 'make a difference', and also that individuals are the single units that make up the whole of society. When we vote, when we chose schools for our children, and sample life styles, we are seen as individuals with the rights and power to be autonomous. However, the thesis of this chapter reminds us of the need to reflect upon what real choices we can make as individuals. In the same way as a child has no choice but to liaise with mental health professionals when considered deviant, we must consider what structures grate against the smooth (M)odern picture of democratic individuality. Practically, this is not hard to do, for when Jill was admitted to the residential unit for her self-harming behaviour, it felt very real to her that she was an individual understood by nobody. The nurses had every intention of respecting her as an individual with unique needs, but they had nursed 'self-harmers a million times'; they even took in the holistic nature of her past, which was entirely unique to her. However, philosophically, the story is very different and seemingly more complex. The two most common theories of epistemological individuation, that is what we know about being individuals, identify spatiotemporal location and the features of substances as their individuators. We know a thing to be individual by its location in space and time or by its features. What this broadly translates to, in practice, is a notion that individuals as contained entities have a relationship with the systems in which they are located. For nursing, this represents the being who is cared-for as another. The nurse caring for Jill will view this care from a holistic framework. However, a major methodological controversy concerns holism versus individualism. Holism maintains that (at least some) social groups must be studied as aggregates, which will not be reducible to their members. Jill's self-harming behaviours automatically frame her within a group exhibiting similar self-harming behaviours. This linking to wider classifications is holist in principle, but has a very delicate relationship with the other important aim of individualising care for Jill. As noted by Rizzo *et al* (1986: 78), 'Epidemics of suicidal attempts are common on an adolescent ward for girls' and, as noted by the postmodernist thinker, Michael (1990: 76), 'the defining parameters of postmodernism in social psychology make plain the overt political purpose of changing prevailing conceptions of the human being [individuality] and the social world'. It is said that the modernist individual is self controlled, unitary, discrete, orderly, orientated towards thought, language, and representation. The postmodern is 'uncontrolled, decentred, multiplicitous, transgressive, orientated towards affect, image, and simulation' (Michael, 1990: 77).

If we attempt to place that which is philosophical to one side or frame it temporarily, it is possible to see that nursing has a tradition which accommodates the Gemeinschaft tradition of holism. Nursing literature advocates the need to view ontology (study of existence) and nursing care as requiring an epistemology, which shares and borrows from the constructivist paradigm. The individual is thus seen as a whole entity, existing at both an intrapersonal and interpersonal level. Individuals are the fundamental unit from which groups of individuals are made. Reduction is thus made possible via systems analysis in this model, which is, itself, supportive of the interpersonal and humanistic approach advocated as being central to all nurse-patient interaction. Individuality not only identifies existence, but is existence. At present, in all the tiers of child and adolescent mental health services (CAMHS), reductionism of individuality has the aim of locating a diagnosis, a deviant label. The diagnosis does not directly consider the unique individuality of the young person's mental health experiences, rather it justifies society's ambiguity and fear about the supposedly broken individual, and licences the concern that leads to intervention (Holyoake, 1998c; 1998d).

As such a broken individual, Jack's (at 14 years old) depression and withdrawn behaviour increased as he found himself in a Tier 4 unit. He had no way of understanding his feelings of low self worth. He was told quite categorically that 'he was depressed' and that 'his feelings of sadness were not natural'. His only way to demonstrate personal authority was to 'beat the illness'. In his own experience, he had felt like this for so long that it felt 'very natural'. The care he received was, therefore, based upon the assumption that, as such a young individual, he was unaware of the 'good times to come'. The assumption was that professional knowledge derived from others' life experiences legitimised treating him. The assignment of a label or a cause pleased his parents and put paid to another assumption (that past events in his life needed to be 'confessed') so that he might progress along a linear scale to full recovery of health, one of the prime goals of individual autonomy.

The assumption that individual experiences reported by young people while receiving care are value-free is a product of the wider discourses located in psychiatry. A central premise of this chapter is to emphasise that there is no possibility of a value-free experience. As noted in previous chapters, 'The Death of the Author' is a postmodernist term that can be used to describe the way young people interact with the processes in which they are involved. The words, concepts, and language we use as nurses (and sometimes as they are used by young people) are loaded with metaphysical assumptions regarding psychiatry and the individual. There may be nothing wrong with this fact, but it would be wilfully wrong to ignore it. The reductionism of positivism is reflected by both humanism and holism, which utilise a similar framework of language to categorise illness. The underlying feature of humanist psychotherapy is a concern with client-centeredness or person-centeredness, that is, the individual as an autonomous being. When considering these issues, it becomes apparent that nursing care is unable to provide all these freedoms; at best, it can only be described as being pseudo humanist because of the constraints placed upon practitioners to ensure safety and professional standards. However, it seems to be the optimism provided by humanism that helps allow it to survive and sit more easily with the labelling of young people, because it attempts to reinforce the faith in values of endurance, nobility, intelligence, and acceptance.

Authority

Plato wrote as a moral absolutist who thought that moral knowledge was 'coded' in the universe. Ethical absolutism like this assumes a bureaucratic model of what morality should be like—a special knowledge known only to experts. Plato assumes that the morality of the individual and the morality of the state are the same thing, (as noted by Martin Pursey (1998)—because there was an obligation on the citizen to participate in the state actively, notably in doing justice). In this respect, his view does not argue well for nursing, as it expresses a determinist and anti-humanist perspective. When claims are made that the state confers authority upon 'experts' to assess and administer care for the good of society (e.g. to put in hospital those who are viewed in the eyes of the world as deviant), it becomes clear that authority is linked to moral attitudes about what to do for the best. A common question nurses ask themselves is, 'Is it in the best interests of the child?' Similarly, Aristotle proposed a humanistic view that everything is heading towards its own unique proper destiny, that human beings and their lives have ascertainable purposes and that it is up to people to realise their full potential. Sensible people do this by choosing a 'mean' between extremes. Perhaps what we are heading towards is 'reasonableness'. Perhaps this is the best we can hope for as nurses. Because authority places a responsibility on individual practitioners to determine the outcomes of practice, authority determines not only the nature of nurse-child interaction, but sets the agenda for those individuals involved. If every individual is unique then no-one can generalise about 'human nature'. It may be that moral philosophy cannot be derived from a definition of human nature, be it having a purpose (Aristotle), or being rational (Kant), or existing as an organism responsive only to pains or pleasures (Bentham). The contemporary belief is that it is we, ourselves, who are ultimately responsible for our essential characters, our nature, and the authority acquired or licenced by our own endeavour. Perhaps it is worth pondering upon the thought that many people have a fear of too much existential freedom, and they seek personal and political authority and domination by others—even if that is at the high moral cost of not living authentically.

Today, postmodernism questions the certainty of a (M)odernism that has graded, labelled, and systematised all our lives and offers us only uncertainty and variety, exemplified in the spectacle of consumerism. The crucial role of the ideological superstructure in manufacturing, the consent of ordinary people to their own oppression appears to be a common Neo-Marxist explanation of why people are not free and accede to authority. Marcuse (1982) explained how capitalism forces people to see themselves primarily as one dimensional isolated consumers with false needs. Capitalist states produce closed forms of discourses so that alternative views are made virtually inexpressible, hence unrealisable. Barthes (1957) uses the term 'myths', adopted in relevant places throughout this book, to describe ideological constructs that parade as being 'natural'. For example, the notion that nurses and organisation naturally form hierarchical structures because this is rational and ordered, as is nature. However, in cheerful contrast, the postmodern vision allows practitioners to invent their own discourses, opposed to the universal truths suggested by large scale moral truths and Utopian visions. It is an existential or Nietzschean vision in which the individual is on a continual quest for self-enrichment and self-enlargement in a world of relative values. In contrast, advanced practice is a (M)odernist project, which aims to produce moral freedoms, authority, and responsibilities that are mainly laced with bizarre optimism. In this respect, it is pro specialist and promotes the vision of 'Neo-tribes' (specialisms) which, unlike traditional tribes (whose authority is based on coercion and hereditary power), would consist of voluntary members who share certain values and have a tribal identity based on self-identification. Hence, the perception that patient care is ultimately best improved within specialist units by specialist and advanced practitioners. Thus, it is assumed that authority is both a personal construct (related to how an individual practitioner perceives personal power) and ability to make a difference, that is, a nurse with authority (i.e. one whose words, instructions, care plans are authoritative) will be more effective with her young patients; a difference that has to take into account the larger structures of unit hierarchy, grade, experience, and personal relationships with other professional colleagues. The hierarchical structures of psychiatry regarding young people emphasises the importance of strict definition and diagnosis.

How one defines illness is part of one's belief system and is largely determined by one's culture. When Jill cuts herself, her behaviour is classified as a disease. However, diseases are abnormalities in the structure and function of body organs and systems and, thus, are a problem of biological malfunctioning. Illness, one the other hand, is perhaps used as a better description, but has to be considered with caution. When Jill describes her feeling of release and control when she cuts, it conjures up concepts of illness because she describes the subjective experience, which is open to expert interpretation. She is seen as sick because her behaviour is perceived and experienced by the larger social group as being abnormal. Whether Jill considers herself well or ill is a matter for experts to deliberate, regardless of her personal ontological experiences. Her symptoms are easily detected as being deviant to the norm, thus necessitating her legitimised loss of freedom and personal choice. It is likely that such behaviour in medieval Europe would have been described as having a supernatural cause, such as witchcraft.

Containment

There is an assumption among nurses caring for children and young people that authority is demonstrated in practice by firmly confronting anti-social behaviours. It is known that a large number of children are referred to child and adolescent mental health services because their behaviour is out of control at home or school. Disruptive problems are seen more often in boys than in girls, with ratios ranging from 4 to 1 to 12 to 1 (American Psychiatric Association, 1987). As noted by Clunn (1991: 234), the chief complaints include: aggressiveness towards others, for example, hitting, kicking and fighting; physical destructiveness; disobedience; and temper tantrums. For adolescents, the behaviours may include rejection of authority, dangerous behaviours to self (cutting, overdoses, drug use), or dangerous behaviour to others (fire setting, violence). Although many medical diagnoses aim to justify and legitimise treatment with terms, such as conduct disorder, attention deficit, and oppositional defiant disorders, such labelling does not provide a framework for nursing care. There is no general consensus regarding strategies for organising nursing care for this type of behaviour. What is apparent is the assumption that a strong sense of authority is seen as curing all ills. This is often heard from staff who say 'it's a lack of boundaries that has turned him/her this way in the first place'. The ability to demonstrate outward authority is seen as a positive characteristic of a nurse, but one that is often described as being the hardest to achieve. In an age that promotes a sense of progress and order, this is hardly surprising. Some nurses speak of learning to be authoritative through experience, watching others. Thus, it seems to be a very haphazard process that raises much anxiety. Nurses working with young inpatients contemplate procedures to prevent outbursts before they occur, raise their own personal profile by being the most confrontational, or legitimise fighting fire with fire by writing specific instructions in care plans. Authority in the containment sense is manifested as **behaviour** that can be quantified and legitimised by the child, and by nursing colleagues.

When to be visible in authority

It is usually held appropriate to display open authority when individual children and young people are involved in anti-social behaviours outside the norm. Quay and Peterson (1984) identify 15 of these behaviours, which include: fights, temper tantrums, disobedience, destructive, attention seeking, dominating others, stealing. These are in no order of severity and the remaining eight behaviours appear to be contentious even for the authors, for their adjectives include: impertinent, uncooperative, disruptive, negative, restless, boisterous, irritable, lies. In order to explore the (M)odernist position regarding authority in more depth, it is necessary to re-visit some of the theories and models that claim to understand authority and, at the same time, legitimise its existence.

The opposite to anti-social behaviour is pro-social behaviour. It includes: altruistic and helping behaviour, routine courtesies, and co-operation. Such behaviour is seen as a normative standard, which is the responsibility of the individual. Children, as they pass through transitional stages, and are socialised by parents, teachers, and others to acquire these values, are encouraged to utilise them for their own advantage and that of others. It has always been thought that children generally behave co-operatively, otherwise they are labelled disruptive or anti-social. Conclusions are drawn as to why a child behaves anti-socially. Perhaps she/he has learnt it from anti-social carers; it may have a biological aetiology; perhaps it is arousal or environmental factors, or a combination of many factors.

In order to understand how children and adolescents perceive authority, we argue (in contrast to the emphasis placed upon checklist assessments by other texts) that these assessment processes are methods to understand patients and get into their world. Assessment tools are just part of the way of being there in caring. The world of the adolescent in psychiatric services is often full of anger, resentment, and self-loathing. Therefore, it comes as no surprise that resistance to psychiatric treatment processes is, itself, labelled (Parker *et al*, 1995), so much so that structural and Post-modern theories view the role of psychiatry as re-educating/re-training individuals into the ways of conformity and compliance expected by families and society. The unique and advanced role of the nurse continues to break this perception via holistic practice, but obedience to authority is often seen as being necessary for 'the child's own good'.

This perception is a legacy of long standing beliefs about authority and development held by experts. In 1946, Flemming (p199) said, 'Adolescent attitudes towards life as a whole differ [to adults]...' He cites Reeves (1946) who discusses the modern youth, and states:

> '1. *The natural world exists solely to be exploited by men. Smash and grab is the only law;*
>
> 2. *The happiest person is he who has the most material possessions; the chief satisfaction in life is to get and get, more and more;*
>
> 3. *The law of the world is competition; the only sensible way to act is to get on, climb up, and push someone else down;*
>
> 4. *Work is a nuisance to be avoided by every device possible; the further up the tree you climb the less work you do, whilst the 'big toff' at the top of the tree does no work at all;*
>
> 5. *The powers that rule this world—known as 'they'—are untrustworthy and arbitrary, to be tricked and outwitted as often, and obeyed as seldom as possible.'*

As noted by MP, this parody-view of adolescents (in an insubordinate post-war world) echoes the middle class moral panic about the bolshie workers' attitude to life reflected in 1950s' and early 1960s' contemporary sociology descriptions (by graduate journalists earning £50–60K) of the excluded underclass. These attitudes sketch a picture of adolescents being hostile towards authority due to their own experience, which often include feelings of inadequacy, anger, a sense of failure, and rejection. The idea that authority can play a role in remedying the isolation and doom perceived by young people is a widespread one. Much emphasis has always been placed upon its use, with little empirical data to support its usefulness. In fact, in general, it has been recognised by nurses that under dictatorial environments young people work submissively and show defiance once supervision is slackened. The adolescent, in his struggle to achieve freedom from his family, often threatens, within himself and his parents, very primitive fears of object loss and separation from symbiotic involvements (Williams, 1986: 180).

Under laissez-faire discipline, adolescents often hunger for direction and support. Therefore, the therapeutic use of self by nursing staff is seen to be the way to utilise authority, doing so within the confines of the caring relationship. The ideal is an interpersonal relationship that values the commitment of both parties and results, over time, in conformity, obedience, and compliance.

These three concepts are widely explored within the paradigm of psychology and social sciences. Conformity is seen as yielding to others, to group pressure, and producing a change in opinions and behaviours, such as, respect for property and a regard for truth. Compliance, however, is the act of doing what you are told without changing your thinking. Obedience is responding to an explicit request, such as, being ordered to make a bed or go to school. Therefore, it can be seen that visual displays of authority are usually within the domain of testing obedience and compliance. The true art of creative nursing care belongs firmly in generating conformity. Authority, in this respect, is ascertainable only in terms of changed behaviour of the young person over a period of time; it does not consist of authoritarian bursts of command and instructions fired off by a nurse under adolescent 'attack'. It is the caring that changes thinking; authority allows for this to happen. The concepts of leaders, power, and norms are important in explaining the process of conformity, obedience, and compliance.

Metaphysics of authority

Is there some truth in the belief that authoritarian parents or carers create first, a dependence and then a rebellious child/young person? According to Herbert (1988), the answer is yes, 'Restrictive, authoritarian parents attempt to shape, control, and assess the behaviour and attitudes of the child according to a set standard of conduct'. It is important to distinguish between that authority which turns into bullying and that which is done with good intention. The difficulty is that the line between them can be very thin. How often do we hear the statement: 'It's for his own good'? The children with authoritarian parents often lack self-confidence, as the controlling authority is a rejection of the child. The child is unable to think, feel, or behave authentically which, taken to extremes, comprises of emotional abuse. On the other hand, permissiveness on the part of parents/carers is just as detrimental, leading to children's demands being met without parents helping children understand or meet the externally defined standards expected by society. This balancing act is at the core of the problem of authority. When does too much authority become detrimental to care? In the past, many nurses have cringed as an authoritarian colleague has scolded a child. Times are changing, legislation provides a framework for protecting the interests of young people in care and identifying responsibilities of nurses (The Children Act, 1989) regarding punitive practice.

The postmodern perspective is that most psychological theory views excessive authority as detrimental. It certainly does not fit into the holistic, humanist model of nursing. As noted by Clark and Gournay (1995: 49), there are a number of 'fairly robust psychological theories' which can improve the understanding of health and health related behaviours essential for the delivery of individualised holistic care. These include: 1) Personal control and learned helplessness; 2) Attribution theory; 3) Information/exchange theory; and 4) The health belief model. Each has the individual as the basis for health and, hence, their importance in the context of individual choices and individualised nursing care. The notion of individual freedom is inseparable from the aim of a patient taking control of his or her life, and responsibility for it. These theories are briefly outlined and will be familiar to most of our readers

However, the (M)odernist view is one that needs to be criticised in order to expose the way interactions between nurses and young people are guided by their hidden assumptions. What are these hidden assumptions? Does it follow that they are similar to those just noted above by Reeves (1946)? If we, as individuals, construct a reality which is based upon such bad premises, it is not that difficult to locate the hidden metaphysics that guide nurses' values regarding authority.

Clark and Gournay (1995: 49) emphasise the effects of 'a belief in self-determination on behaviour' regarding the theory of personal control. The idea of self-determination or agency can be defined as the belief that individuals have control over what happens to them. The lack of this idea leads to people perceiving that they have no mastery over present and future events, and (for our purposes) a reduction of purposeful action to influence personal outcomes of health. The theoretical underpinning of this health psychology is the way people learn and think, and the most applicable theory is social learning theory. We, as individuals, exist without justification in a world into which we are thrown, condemned to assume full responsibility for our free actions and for the very values according to which we act. This is the Sartrean ontology of Being and nothingness (Sartre, 1990).

Social learning theory evolved from traditional behavioural theory, the major component being the positivist notion of mechanical cause and effect; that is, a person's behaviour is always affected by the consequences of previous behaviours. The work of B F Skinner (1938) in operant learning theory emphasises the importance of two concepts in behaviourism. First, reinforcement—the result of a consequence which is rewarding and pleasurable or the avoidance of unpleasant experiences. (As described in many textbooks, the process of reinforcement involves either applying a positive stimulus (positive reinforcement) or removing an unpleasant one (negative reinforcement)). The second important concept is punishment used to prevent or extinguish behaviour. Social learning theory is best known due to the work of Bandura (1986). His theories emphasise the importance of thinking, as well as the importance of reinforcement and punishment. In this way, social learning theory fills the empty 'black box' of behaviourism, which has traditionally neglected anything that cannot be measured in terms of behaviour. As noted by Clark and Gournay (1995: 51), the study of mental processes that are involved in making sense of the environment (such as perception, learning, memory, language, problem-solving and thinking) 'had largely developed in isolation from operant learning theory'. The importance of social learning theory with regard to the development of children cannot be under-estimated. Imitation by children and the effects of modelling are central to the theories of Bandura, and emphasise the active part people play in their interaction with their world. In theory, children are seen to learn through being conditioned, as reacting to various sets of stimuli, such as positive reinforcement. However, as noted by Clark and Gournay (1995: 52), such a view contrasts with the belief held by many that we can make our own decisions about how we act, and that we exert considerable control over our behaviour.

Attribution theory is broadly about understanding why people behave the way that they do. The work of Heider (1958) emphasises the human need to know why others behave in a specific way. People attribute reasons for others' behaviour, if they lack an explanation, or find a given explanation unsatisfactory. The process of trying to understand can be divided into two notions of attribution. First, internal factors, which relate to the person or individual. This is the personal experiences, memories, and cognitive abilities of the individual. Second, external factors that relate to the situation an individual finds him/herself in at any particular moment.

Conclusion

It is supposed throughout this chapter that nurses have a privileged, powerful position over the young people they nurse. It is also supposed that the nature of individuality is a concept central to the debate about notions of authority and autonomy. As such, the idea that an individual young person has automatic political and/or social emancipation can be seen to reflect the traditional model of linear progression that underlies (M)odernism. The idea that individuals will somehow be liberated in the future is a grand myth as each progressive set of ideas transcends the previous set. This scepticism towards the grand narratives of what authority and individuality actually constitutes in child and adolescent mental health nursing is a function of the knowledge base adopted by the dominant paradigm at any point in time. Today, in nursing and society generally, knowledge can be viewed as a post-industrial force of production. The important notion, as noted by Appignanesi and Garratt (1995: 106), at the core of this chapter is, 'What's new [about this postmodern age] is the production of a completely new type of knower.' The parents, the young people, and the health professionals as individuals have a pragmatic knowledge that has ceased to be an end in itself. No longer, in this world of hyper, cyber, and simulated experience, can knowledge of the individual just be assumed to be encompassed in a set of narratives devoid of time and place. The individual authority issues discussed throughout this chapter identify the belief that authority is used to re-normalise and reinforce moral judgements reflected by society at large. This postmodern view presents a hyper-surreal view of a detached authority, which is experienced at an individual level by a young person, as being personal and necessary to instigate individual change in a world that is far detached from the natural reality it simulates.

Nursing staff comments

'When I first started nursing adolescents I found it really difficult to stand up to them…I found myself trying to compromise with them, but my colleagues

thought I was soft. It took me ages to accept that my way was different, and I think that's good, because you need a skill mix don't you?"

'I've seen a few nurses make some really stupid decisions regarding their power. Some of them think they can order the kids around as a God-given right'

'There's definitely a difference between telling a child off and an adolescent… with the adolescent, you have to be more in tune with what's going on for them rather than the immediate problem behaviour'

'No, I've never really thought about the broader philosophical issues, such as, legitimacy. I don't think we have time to do that when you're trying to separate two scrapping children who both want the same toy.'

Chapter 10
Milieu and self-care

'The use of the word 'leave' implies that someone has been given permission to go.'

Bayliss (1995: 187)

Dialogue

Dean: There's been a lot of change in mental health provision over the last five years. This includes the HAS report in child and adolescent services, but what intrigues me, is the view nurses have of residential units and their usefulness.

Sandy: Tier 4 services are needed for those young people who are in need of safety, you know, sanctuary from the outside world. Although we know most nursing care can be adequately provided in the community.

Dean: Exactly ! So what do we use residential units and milieu stuff for?

Sandy: I think that it's assumed that they need to exist because of the safety aspect.

Dean: There's a belief that these environments are for the most distressed young people. It is assumed that they provide an environment beyond the physical constraints of bricks and mortar. They provide a therapeutic milieu. This is an accepted assumption which justifies their existence. Linked to this is the idea that the existence of mental illness in young people ensures their existence.

Sandy: And our jobs...

Dean: No doubt. As nurses we justify our role by controlling the milieu and advocating a self care ethos which is fundamentally impossible. We remove the risk from society at large and place it firmly on the shoulders of the individual.

Sandy: So what are you saying?

Dean: I'm saying that we need to write something about these assumptions to get the debate going...at least I think that's what I'm saying.

Thesis for this chapter

- ❑ The principle of self-care is a smoke screen, which attempts to overcome the difficulty that patients are and always will be in a less powerful position
- ❑ The use of therapeutic milieu as a clinical intervention assumes that a miniature reflection of the modern society that is said to have contributed to illness can, in some way, be part of its solution. It is a (M)odernist blunder inspired by a truly modern lack of thought.

Background and aims

This chapter argues that the milieus of most residential child and adolescent units in the UK share common characteristics. A central assumption is that the milieu is an important prerequisite of the care process and, as such, provides structures and processes that can help shape and predict care outcomes. These outcomes are seen as a result of Tier 4 provision rather than the result of care at home or in the community. As such, the decision to use the residential unit (which is usually seen as the last resort) is an attempt at manipulating the inpatient environment to promote health. The development of milieu as a therapeutic tool has also been a recognition of the way humans form natural collectives, be it for safety, extended security, or survival. As noted by Thornbory and Murugiah, (1995: 29), Einstein is reputed to have said that the environment is everything that is not me; others have said that the environment is everything including me. The latter is based upon the Hiedeggarian phenomenological perspective. There have been countless textbooks citing many theories, all claiming to have the answer to why animals, primates, and humans group together. The theories fill a wide a spectrum from biological anthropology to psychoanalysis. However, these theories are not the primary concern of this chapter, which instead aims to critically explore two central issues related to the milieu provided by Tier 4 institutions. First, the question of what milieu actually is. It is argued that the milieu provided by Tier 4 institutions is artificial and not defensible as a therapeutic process in which children and young people are nursed, in order to provide an opportunity for them, as individuals, to be exposed to others, and to relate to them as a prelude to wider society. In short, 'milieu' presupposes using other patients as therapy. Second, we pose the fundamental issue of self-care as the ultimate care objective. It is argued that self-care is a nursing ideology that can never be fulfilled per se, certainly not within an institutional setting, and one that is rarely necessary in child and adolescent health. This chapter contemplates the hidden assumptions and issues related to closed environments and the desire for an intensive, total therapy. Its basic concern being first, the speculative and opportunistic nature of a therapy, which is part of a psychiatric ideology dominated by diagnosis, classifications, and predictable outcomes. The second concern is the nature of the nurse-young person interface or interaction within a rigid and unrelenting environment and subject to such positivist procedures as the nursing process.

Aims

1. To provide a brief outline of what milieu is thought to be;
2. To explore the issues that are oppressive to the milieu Utopia; and
3. To explore issues related to the concept of self-care.

Assuming the consequences of an environment

As a prelude to the theory of milieu therapy, the authors feel it is important to bear in mind that milieu therapy is not the same as managing an environment or culture. It encompasses many differing philosophical issues. Again, environments can be as harmful as they can be beneficial. The literature regarding the care of children and young people clearly demonstrates a belief that the environment, and the management of it, can be used effectively as a therapeutic tool. Some even consider it as important as the therapeutic use of self—a belief that the environment is more potent than the people in it creating change—as noted by Pasquali *et al* (1989: 343), 'In addition to relationship therapy, the nurse who works in a psychiatric setting is usually involved in important elements of milieu therapy'. Such is the supposed importance of milieu that Steinberg (1987: 248) states, 'The pressures of social groups, both to explore feelings and attitudes and to help modify them, are important components in a wide variety of group and social therapies'. The assumption that the environment can be managed to provide the social therapy for hospitalised young people is a considered assumption, according to which the opportunity to include a young person is not only beneficial, but even desirable. It is supposed to be beneficial because of the artificial manipulation of an environment that aims to be non-artificial and be a miniature version of wider society. In short, it should be something which is 'normal'. So, there seem to be two distinct issues related to what occurs in practice and what is seen to be beneficial in theory.

Simply managing the environment is not milieu therapy. For example, attempting to control stimuli and unit routines does not provide a natural milieu attempted by, say, a therapeutic community. In fact, environmental manipulation has specific objectives, which serve to provide containment and order. These may be seen as qualities expected in society. They are qualities which are imposed by man over nature in a supposedly evolutionary way. As noted by Hoare (1993: 174), most advice given to teachers and parents about changes in a child's routine or overall environment may include: 'placement of the child in a small, stable teaching group, time limitation for individual activities, alterations to classroom layout, careful controls of the number of activities'. As such, these instructions reflect the routines of most residential units. For example, the times of meals and medicine rounds, set groups with set members, specific activities on set days at set times, and the allocation of free time, which young people are actively encouraged to spend constructively. Brown and Clunn (1991: 448) note that therapeutic milieu strategies 'foster communication, problem-solving, ego-enhancement and socialisation'. Therefore, it seems there is little doubt that residential environments can provide therapeutic milieu and that a therapeutic milieu is beneficial. However, this assumes that communication is a good thing or that ego-enhancement is, metaphysically, a stable concept. The extent to which a residential environment can provide a therapeutic milieu needs exploring.

The history of therapeutic milieu

The idea that the environment has an effect upon humans is an old assumption. It can be seen clearly in the constructions of the ancient world, such as, the temples and tombs built by man for gods and kings. The grand nature of the pyramids and Hanging Gardens of Babylon inspired awe and exceeded the mere substance of these wonders of the ancient world. They were succeeded by bigger and more complex cathedrals and other buildings, which aimed to inspire and denote a greatness in the supernatural beliefs of their time. As noted by Pasquali *et al* (1989: 344), 'Milieu is the French word for middle or middle place: in English we use it to mean environment'. It demonstrates the belief that conditions can act as an agent or a middle medium to stir emotions in man. The idea of a therapeutic milieu has a more recent history that was born from the notion of 'moral management. As noted by Nolan (1993: 42), 'caring for the insane was partly due to an awakening of public consciousness and partly to a new spirit of management'. This new spirit also proclaimed the separation of childhood and the emergence of adolescence from adulthood as a transitionary period. Indeed, the attempt to control the environment for particular categories of mental patients went hand in hand with the moral movements at the turn of the century. The increased opposition to mechanical restraints reflected liberalism and an increased acceptance that mental illness was a biological reality, rather than idleness or a spiritual manifestation. The idea that the milieu could be therapeutic emphasised the practical difficulties of abolishing physical means of restraint and, as noted by Nolan (1993: 43), 'seclusion and solitary confinement had often to replace it ...private madhouses brought into use padded cells for violent patients'.

On a broader scale, the need for asylums to provide safety for the public at large reflects the power, which the state and the discourses of psychiatry has over the individual. This power is based upon moral philosophical claims which, today, are softened by humanistic interventions by care staff. The claim that a therapeutic milieu should install an ethos of shared work, responsibility, and regularity still echoes from the Victorian asylum system, which operated as a self-contained unit. The difference is that, nowadays, therapeutic communities are supposed to be preparing young people for life in wider society outside of the milieu. The young person enters the 'middle' (milieu) in a moral transaction, which partly involves preparing and practising for reunion with society and himself. In Victorian times, the treatment milieu lacked this intention almost entirely. Indeed, as understood by Nolan (1993: 96), it was not until the introduction of the Mental Treatment Act in 1930 that asylums formally became hospitals. It was not until the passing of the Act that the concept of mental disorder as illness was cautiously accepted (Jones, 1991: 25). Thus began the notions of madness and abnormal psychology as we understand them today in the UK. As noted by Parker *et al* (1995: 1), these notions are 'particular and peculiar to our culture and our time', a time in which it is widely assumed by authority that child and adolescent residential units provide an environment of normality and therapeutic milieu. However, the young people are forced into fitting a diagnosis and all too often compelled to enter a residential clinic (or unit), given no alternative by parents and concerned professional experts. Analytical minds of the modern era created a certain knowledge about modern social problems. As argued by Foucault (1971), the recorded increases in the number of the insane and the heavier burdens of the asylum programme became an emotive symbol of what industrial progress and city life had done to the natural fabric. The idea that even children were affected by illness drew upon the statistical evolution of sociology, which played an important part in sustaining the myth that mental illness really existed and needed confronting with institutions. The cases of injustice towards patients and the need to humanise therapeutic environments (be they smaller non-hierarchal ones advocated by psychiatrists, such as the pioneer R D Laing) will always remain an issue, but the certainty remains that communities of an institutional kind disempower individuals. Masson (1990: 243) argues that humanistic principles, such as those noted by Rogers and Stevens (1971), do not give any sense of what it is like for patients living in these oppressive environments. Indeed, these environments are most certainly more hostile than a caring family environment in the experience of most young people (except for those who have never experienced secure object relational attachments).

Underlying assumptions

Maxwell Jones (1953), a Scottish psychiatrist, developed a treatment modality not unlike that advocated by the HAS Report (1995). He sought a modality that uses the environment—its physical facilities, various therapies, and interpersonal relationships—to foster a healthy personality (Pasquali *et al*, 1989). The community serves as a container in which residents learn to be social and grow interpersonally at their own pace. The community becomes a small-scale reflection of society with specific community constructs. The interpersonal becomes more personal as each member of the community is actively encouraged to confront others, in contrast to wider society where we generally employ other paid professionals, such as solicitors. In such miniature communities, staff have to play a dual role as the cost of membership. They are equal citizens, but also police and guards. As noted by Pasquali *et al*, (1989: 344), Jones outlined what he saw as five basic principles of a therapeutic community :

1. Responsibility for treatment belongs not only to physician and staff but also to the residents;

2. Social distance between staff and residents is reduced; this may permit free discussion of the behaviour of staff members as well as the behaviour of residents;
3. A democratic atmosphere is cultivated;
4. Open communication in the form of shared feelings and information is strongly encouraged; and
5. Deviant behaviour is controlled and social learning takes place through the mechanism of resident-staff meetings.

The HAS Report's (1995) general premise argues for the increased growth of specialist knowledge and creative development of services. However, the plausibility of hospital units becoming therapeutic communities, as advocated by the above principles, is very slight. What is striking about these principles, however, is their humanistic qualities. It is argued that it is this humanism that allows many nurses to consider their practice in the context of therapeutic milieu. As such, young people are encouraged to take responsibility in their own care, but not for the organisation of the unit. Personal interaction is seen as an opportunity to communicate, educate, teach, and experience human closeness. Active participation is seen to offer opportunities to test out control and autonomy, and peer pressure as a way to experience the needs of others. The use of treatment within the boundaries of mainstream theory is utilised in non-directional informal settings. These include art, writing, pottery, music, individual, and group therapy. In such ways, the setting is operationalised to provide a therapeutic milieu within the confines of medical, expert, and specialised structures. In an era that seems to be highlighting the fragmented nature of individuality, and the need to promote increased self-care and individualised care planning, the objectives of therapeutic milieu would appear to be a thorny issue. The functionalist use of peer pressure to determine another individual's care, the need for agendas, graded responsibilities, roll call, albeit within an optimistic philosophy, does not rest comfortably with the recommendations of the HAS Report (1995) or with individual care. These criticisms serve only to warn us that a therapeutic milieu requires vast input and resources in order to produce long lasting outcomes. Most Tier 4 services are not able to provide this.

Criticising milieu as therapy

Consider the passage below. Note its sentiments and metaphysical assumptions because, broadly speaking, it incorporates all that we, as nurses, take for granted regarding milieu and Tier 4 residential units :

> *'If a psychiatrist had not deemed you mentally ill in the first place there would be no need for you to be grateful for this milieu therapy, because you wouldn't be in it. But as it is obvious that mental illness in young people and childhood exists, then we have to thank God that the walls are thick and that they can contain the madness' (Musing by Dean, 1998).*

Perhaps it could be argued that better multi-disciplinary assessment would stop inappropriate referrals (what ever they are) being admitted, or, as often overheard in nursing offices through out the UK, the misuse of diagnostic criteria can only be the fault of medics. By analysing the deep assumptions, such as those in the above passage, we can begin to understand the metaphysical philosophical issues. First, it is always assumed that mental illness exists. We assume that it does, because little John (6 years of age) continually swears and hits his younger sister. Perhaps there is a biological explanation, perhaps it is his diet, or his lack of appropriate parenting. We know that mental illness exists because big John (14 years of age) is easily distracted, has poor concentration, and appears to laugh at something no one else can see. It is obvious that help is needed. We need a doctor, a doctor of the mind not the body. The psychiatrist knows that the two lads are mad because he's seen it all before and, after all, he is a consultant psychiatrist so why else is his time and attention being sought. Phew, is he glad that there are Tier 4 provisions for these two, because things are getting out of hand. Luckily, he's the one with the power in society to remove the two boys from circulation, so that everyone can breath a sigh of relief. The nurses in the unit have also seen it all before. Little John doesn't like to be told off and has a tantrum, while mom hopes that a biological cause can be found. Meanwhile big John's parents are also hoping a biological cure can be found. The nurses defend the psychiatric diagnosis, because they and their workplace have to proceed on the assumption that mental illness exists. These walls will keep everyone safe until the natural madness has gone away. To help this happen, the two will be forced to attend groups, criticise and be criticised by others, have limited privacy, and be expected to 'toe the line'.

Although this scenario should be read tongue in cheek, it highlights the general experience that most Tier 4 provision is usually the end of the line. Health care professionals work with young people to ensure they are able to return home after acute or chronic illness (we mean, of course, an illness which might not even exist). But supposing a young person is distressed? Surely it cannot be possible to argue that distress is healthy and perhaps not an illness that needs specialised input? The fact that humans feel and exhibited a range of emotions, be they happy or sad, is a phenomenon outside psychiatry. Psychiatry does not have the monopoly on how young people should feel. To comfort patients by offering a diagnosis does not make the social realities of wider society any better. It just reinforces the power base that psychiatry has. For example, psychiatry has the ability to create sickness, which determines if parents are able to claim expenses, benefits, or other support. Psychiatry makes the diagnosis that promotes a sick role, which disempowers and disables young people by making them believe that they are not normal, well, or worthy to take their place in society. As noted by Wood (1983) in his book The Myth of Neurosis, the uses of psychiatry just reinforce 'talk therapy and tranquillisers [which] damage self-respect and sustain the illness excuse'. However, finding the ability to change a system and powerful discourse, such as psychiatry, is an overwhelming task, one that is not to be achieved by individuals, or by theorists alone. Therefore, this book proposes the deconstruction of psychiatry metaphysically to emphasise that there are alternative views to this dominant discourse, which is perceived as being the protector of all those experiencing 'mental health' and as a persecutor to those suffering 'mental illness'.

Our changing perceptions of mental health and mental illness dictate a re-evaluation of Tier 4 inpatient services; in particular, we must think about what we expect them to achieve. If we view mental illness as a biological phenomenon (and this is being challenged more and more), then any changes in institutional care in the long term will undoubtedly be in terms of economic preference. The paradigm of nursing, if consistent with a holistic and constructivist perspective, has to acknowledge that institutional care in terms of milieu therapy is, at present, the best we can offer as a solution to the wider societal issues of madness. It is acknowledged that nurses carry the greatest responsibility for maintaining a safe and secure environment within Tier 4 services. Their role is interwoven with other members of the multi-disciplinary team, and the need to be co-operative in that role ultimately results in a reluctant acceptance of medical classifications and diagnosis for all young people. From a holistic point of view, there is a natural tendency to focus upon the psychosocial problems of a child, as well as his biological difficulties. However, the responsibilities and accountabilities of team work form part of the usual functionalist structure that decides upon care packages and treatment modalities. The hierarchical and authoritarian nature of team approaches (which is explored in our other chapters) is an anti-thesis to milieu therapy, and tends to work against it in practice. Often the most important team member is asked to contribute last, if at all. Most young people have little say in what structures they encounter, and it is generally held that the nurse's role is one of advocacy rather than fellow community dweller. Therefore, the attempt to provide a pure therapeutic milieu within a hospital/medical Tier 4 setting cannot be achieved. This is not to say that principles of therapeutic milieu cannot be utilised, but the incomplete and partial nature of 'milieu therapy' has to be acknowledged.

According to Fann and Goshen (1977), milieu therapy is 'a therapeutic approach to hospital psychiatry in which the entire hospital environment is designed to facilitate rehabilitation. This includes occupational therapy, recreational therapy, team approach, work assignments, and education of all who work in the hospital and participate in the care of patients' (cited in Pasquali *et al*, 1989). The HAS Report (1995: 99) states that 'inpatient and day patient facilities should not only be used to bring effective therapeutic leverage to bear on severe and otherwise intractable problems, but admission to them should also be considered as a strategic manoeuvre within more comprehensive therapeutic programmes', i.e., the unit milieu alone cannot be relied upon to bring about socially constructed change. Inpatient admission has never been offered by carers as a complete solution to a child's mental health problems, but is always described as a benefit and ultimate solution to safety needs. It is no doubt that the culture of institutional settings does provide opportunities for personal growth and development for many young people. This is explored in other chapters, but the need for individually created care packages, which should always include issues of self-care, is seen as the way forward within all hospital therapeutic milieus. The difficulty arises when you consider the metaphysical foundations upon which milieu therapy and self-care are founded. The two are opposing concepts in that a young person would never be allowed to be totally self-caring, because the regulations which come with the milieu would restrain such a development. It is also likely that the experience of being a psychiatric inpatient—oppressive to many teenagers—will, itself, destroy a youngster's will to progress, to get back to normality. Therefore, as nurses, we contemplate the individual needs of our patients with the knowledge that all residential units can never reflect wider society, because residential units are wider society. In fact, they focus and intensify the demands and aspirations of society, putting the young residents under an arc-light of expectation. The myth of therapy promotes the idea that mental illness can be detached and repaired by experts. It is a powerful discourse to which health professionals unwittingly subscribe. Likewise, the promotion of clinical career pathways for individual nurses provides a mirror reflecting this supposedly needs-led approach. On a broader scale, 'the thinking of local authority purchasers is towards defining managed packages of care, orientated to the assessed needs of children, adolescents and their families' (HAS, 1995: 89). Therefore, residential or Tier 4 services are a secure environment in which care can be delivered systematically, away from harm's way. The environment is one in which nurses attempt to utilise aspects of self-care, in order to promote individuality within a group.

Institutional self-care ethic?

The principles of therapeutic milieu share a common foundation with the holistic and humanist principles derived from kinship and family. The friction caused between the practicalities of milieu and the prized goal of self-care reflects the individualistic/anti-individualistic dichotomy. It emphasises that postmodern thought is a part of a definite epistemological and political break from modernist social psychology. The modern, with its belief that individuals are free (even within the realms of behaviourist determinism) to choose how to act and humanistically choose to live the 'good life', contrasts violently with the postmodern construct of the self-determining subject of modern political, legal, social, and aesthetic discourse. The modernist idea that communities are micro-organisms in a constant state of flux, and have changing dynamics with ages and stages, demonstrates how certain principles can be seen to apply within Tier 4 settings. Reflecting this constant state of flux is the view that 'Health can be viewed as a state of dynamic equilibrium between the individual and his environment' (Hinchliff *et al*, 1993). This view has been called the 'metaphysics of human agency (Fay, 1987: 26). It is 'an inflated conception of the powers of human reason and will' (p9) (cited in Lather, 1990: 102). That attempt to emphasise the ability of young people to create their own choices is opposed by Foucault's (1976) deconstruction, which argues that a privileged centering of concepts is a reduction to single systems of thought, such as the notions of autonomy and free will. The postmodern claim is that the truth is not of our own making, and proposes the 'death of the subject' or individual for analysis in a bid to dismiss key notions of the Enlightenment, such as the Kantian ideal of a moral subject taking the ultimate responsibility for his or her actions. As noted by Lovlie (1990: 131), 'The same holds true for the romantic ideas of a self-creative individual transcending the boundaries of social and political restrictions, as well as for the pragmatic belief in a problem-solving individual aiming at the reconstruction of personal and cultural ideals'. The young patient as an inpatient is part of a select population, one that views itself as being different from the population at large. The differences include labels of mental illness and messages received about the type of environment that defines—or dictates—their health status for them. As such, the inpatient Tier 4 environment has a massive impact upon the individual and his or her family. Indeed, as noted by Thornbory and Murugiah (1995: 34), 'most nursing models mention the environment as part of the human ecosystem'. Such an ecosystem in terms of Tier 4 provision is very artificial and generates a dependency felt by every individual within it. Most nursing models (with their systems orientation) adopt a philosophical position, which determines a positivist cause and effect relationship between nursing's input and its supposed outcomes. Therefore, the attempt to create an environment or milieu, which allows a young person to have control, shared responsibility through action, and legislation may be said to be holistic and humanistic in theory, but those theoretical claims will be hard to verify and, we believe, will not be met in the reality of practice. So how do we improve milieu to ensure its usefulness in attaining practical care outcomes?

The ultimate aim of this chapter is to explore the use of the environment in nursing mentally ill young people and children. It is often assumed that these environments are the most important facet of the service, in terms of providing safety, thus, partly justifying the removal of a child from the family home. The expectation is that such a safe environment will lead to the ultimate in nursing care objectives, that of self-care. As such, the milieu has to allow the child or young person to be involved in all stages of care management. In order to allow this to happen, the approach of the nurse and the flexibility of the milieu is usually tested to the full in order to try and meet these expectations. It is very difficult to re-arrange unit routines, rules, and cultural rituals in order to provide a milieu which fully meets the demands placed upon it. In fact, it is impossible for nursing staff to provide an environment that caters for every individual uniquely, so compromises have to be made. These explain the generally limited nature of self-care programs in Tier 4 provisions. Let us now consider the second assumption, that milieu enables the young person to progress or move forward in order to achieve self-care objectives. In this context, nursing as a process assumes that, where a self-care deficit exists and an individual young person is unable to adapt within the confines of the milieu, then nursing care may be needed. As noted by Bayliss (1995: 184) the goals of nursing 'are to enable individuals to attain their own therapeutic self-care demands'. For nurses working with children and adolescents, this can be viewed as being extremely difficult given the demands of the milieu and the nature of childhood development. Therefore, the authors argue that nursing within this speciality cannot be said to promote a self-care model (as, say, does Orem (1991)), even when one takes into account the nature of the individual, because Tier 4 nurses are confined by the norms of the therapeutic milieu. Self-care and milieu are very much discourses in themselves and are a result of the smothering effects of medicalisation and institutionalisation. As noted by Richer (1990: 115), 'Social systems are characterised by inertia. Change is slow and rarely the result of individual efforts'. As previously argued, the ideologies are self-preserving and serve the dominant discourse of psychiatry. At best, nursing continues in its constructivist holism to loosen some of the screws and deconstruct some of these discourses regarding first, the ability of institutional care to provide an ill-defined notion of what therapeutic institutions are and are capable of, and second, the assumption that self-care is attainable by young people.

What this chapter has attempted to highlight is the need for nurses to question the role Tier 4 services and the management of milieu interventions can really play in the lives of hospitalised children and young people? The fact that self-care initiatives can be seen to belong within the framework of humanist and holistic nursing philosophy does not enable self-care to be an achievable reality for this client group.

It is better to ask the question, 'What level of self-care can this individual reach and function at? Is this milieu able to make that happen? Thus the two mainstream assumptions already highlighted (Tier 4 milieu is beneficial for some young people and Milieu should lead to more independent self-care) can be viewed, not as universal truths, but as possible determinants of Tier 4 use.

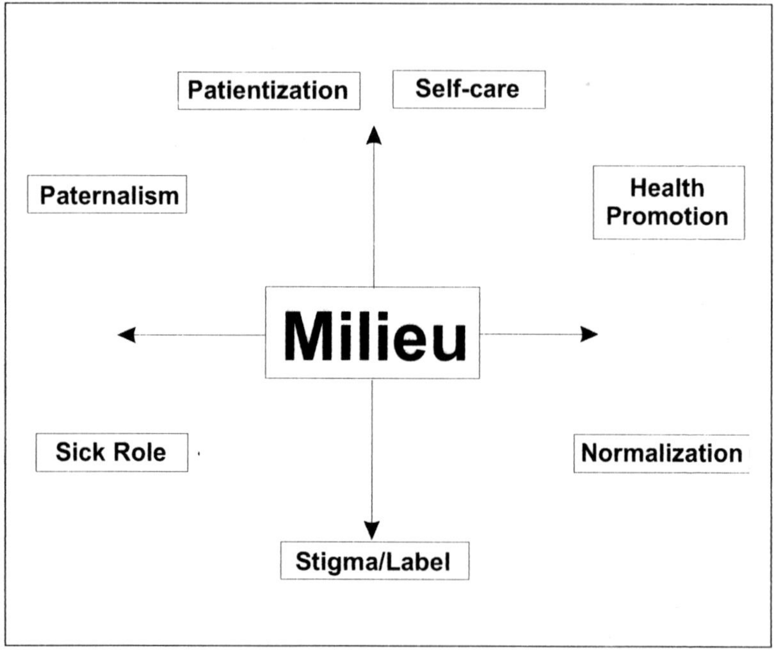

Levin (1981) sees self-care as involving empowerment and encouraging self-reliance in health care (Bayliss, 1995: 187). It is argued that empowering children and young people is not necessarily a high priority issue for nurses in child and adolescent mental health. It would be absurd to believe that a 7-year-old could or even should be empowered to take control and be self-reliant. The real priority is to realise that empowerment as a concept can never be fully achieved because of the powerful discourses that exist in psychiatry. As a romantic notion, empowerment makes nurses feel good about their role as advocate, but it blinds us all into believing that empowerment is actually what we think it is. For example, when we empower a 14-year-old to be more independent, it usually involves the practice of going out more, making decisions about his/her personal time management, and maybe the use of a medi-pack, but the usefulness of such nursing action exists within the paradox that exists within modern nursing practice. The need for more independence will more often be nurse-initiated, motivated, and evaluated, because the dominant discourse is that independence is necessary and good. This is not to say that it is not, but by way of a shallow deconstruction, the authors continue to highlight that such assumptions are not the only ones. They are those which are currently in vogue and culture driven, and palatable to the present day milieu. Perhaps this argument is just a play on words, because it could be argued that this is just an argument for 'needs led' nursing care. The authors would point out that this notion, in itself, is metaphysically and discourse driven. The aim is to deconstruct the foundations of theory rather than just assume. In practice, a young person can be involved in self-care if they and the residential unit understand and jointly own the tenets of patient autonomy, participation, power sharing, full information, and partnership in the care process. Usually, this is not what happens, nor can the necessary changes be made to bring it about.

Young person's comments

John (7)	It's the doctors who will make things better. I know that that's what everyone wants
Sally (13)	There's no point in trying to help yourself in a place like this, because everyone is just treated the same anyway
Susan (15)	When I first came here, I though everyone was like a robot or something, but I don't have to attend every group so that's OK

Last remarks

This chapter has focussed upon the two specific assumptions that enable Tier 4 care provision to have its place within child and adolescent mental health services. It concludes that Tier 4 services aim to provide a milieu that follows the basic tenets of therapy, but is very rarely able to provide individualised care. This has consequences for the philosophy that underlies nursing care. The notion of providing individualised nursing care in an environment, which is clearly dependent upon the collective nature of human groups is, and will always be, fraught with difficulties. These difficulties are highlighted by the assumption that milieu should allow young people to be involved in tailor-made self-care programs, but these conflict with milieu philosophy. The chapter also concludes that self-care is, and will also always remain, the ultimate health care objective, but will never be attained. In this respect, it is a myth and one that is rarely understood, especially in work with young people. In child services, nurses speak of patients learning to be accountable for actions. In adolescent nursing, it is more about patients moving on. The environment works in such a way that it seems to ensure its own existence through the ideology of a dominant discourse.

Section IV: The future Utopia: The new post, postmodern

('Utopia' actually means 'No-place' i.e. cloud cuckoo land and imaginary-ville. It is often used to mean 'Much sought-after [but unachievable] objective'. The word carries too much excess baggage from the history of ideas to be used carelessly. After all, as noted by MP 'we don't mean to imply that "Utopia' is a fantastic or imaginary 'place-to- be'".

Aims for this section

(1) To provide a dialogue which attempts to validate the themes of this book.

(Mark the box(s) for a correct answer, a negative mark for an incorrect answer. More than one may be true)

Q1. Does Tier 4 inpatient culture relate to:

A. ❑ Peer culture, nursing culture, institutionalisation, traditional rituals

B. ❑ Pressure for compliance, attachment and ownership, power, traditional carriers of culture

C. ❑ Goffman, Sartre, Durkheim, Foucault

D. ❑ Determinism, Liberty, The Self

E. ❑ Utilitarianism, existentialism, functionalism, structuralism, postmodernism.

Q2. How would (M)odernist scholars describe the world of mentally ill young people?

A. ❑ Inmate, ritualistic, non-mobile, forced, disculturation

B. ❑ Predictable, isolated, false, ordered, fraternalised

C. ❑ Intrusive, universal, underworld, withdrawn, humiliating

D. ❑ Bureaucratic, policed, public, defensive, privilege system

E. ❑ Full of 'tinkers', guards, officials, concern with 'people work'.

Q3. What is peer culture like when observed?

A. ❑ Accepting, secret, hierarchic, adaptive

B. ❑ Caring, supportive, friendly, honest, character-forming

C. ❑ Regulated, fragmented, evolving, enabling

D. ❑ Power displays, dual incentives, maternalised, inevitable

E. ❑ Self-care, empowered, beneficial, necessary.

Q4. What is the nature of the nursing culture?

A. ❑ Patriarchal, dominant, powerful, ritualistic

B. ❑ Determined, ordered, intrusive, traditional carriers of culture

C. ❑ Universal, evolving, informed, ideologically driven

D. ❑ Technical, clinical, managed, hierarchical

E. ❑ Fordist, pressure for compliance, ruling class, elitist.

Q5. The reason why the peer culture and the dominant nursing culture share so many of Goffman's ad hoc concepts is due, in part, to his descriptive ability. Theorist who have advanced the study of power and culture in contemporary discussion describe this theory as:

A. ❑ Related to Marxist materialism, Foucault's structuralism, Sartre's existentialism

B. ❑ Choice, self-care, advocacy, empowerment

C. ❑ Status, ruling elite, visible and invisible power, objectivity

D. ❑ Consumerism, civil rights, ethics, legitimate

E. ❑ Self-determination, self-actualisation, responsible, sick role.

Q6. The explorative nature of this book cannot be conclusive, but it has attempted to utilise theoretical frameworks familiar from the study of culture. Such frameworks may include:

A. ❑ Anthropology, ethnography, grounded theory, ethnoscience

B. ❑ Descriptive, explorative, naturalistic

C. ❑ 'In the field', native, investigative

D. ❑ Qualitative, interpretative, holistic, contextual

E. ❑ Observation, artefacts, diaries, interviews, belonging.

Q7. What are the main points for reflection highlighted in this book?

A. ❑ Tier 4 services often justify loss of liberty via expert assessment and diagnosis

B. ❑ Dynamics of family life are used to justify admission (medicalizing the problem)

C. ❑ Surveillance is not therapy

D. ❑ Hospitalisation is an old solution in a new world

E. ❑ We are all victims of discourse.

All Answers Are Correct.

Chapter 11
Concluding dialogue (re-thinking the book)

Dean: We set out to contribute something original to child and adolescent mental health nursing... As we said at the start, something post HAS Report, something that touched upon the academic developments of the latter part of the twentieth century, something post-modern.

Sandy: It is important to note that we viewed postmodernism as both a development of, and a result of, modernist epistemology and of which child and adolescent nursing is unavoidably a part.

Dean: The idea of looking back in order to look forward and explore the ideas of 'progress' were our initial motives. The idea of providing a valid alternative frame of reference to the more logical project of Modernist thinking started to unearth ideas that challenged the traditional way we tend to view child and adolescent nursing.

Sandy: I believe we have tried to introduce some of those ideas throughout this book.

Dean: Yes, I think we have; for example, the notion of 'the self' as a constructed identity, which is made up of powerful relationships and cultural influences. Similarly, the idea of continually shifting 'power discourses', which are made up of dialogue and choice. I think that our theses highlight the main ideas of the book.

Sandy: The first being that one does not have to scratch too far below the surface to understand that struggles about ideology, power, and knowledge are inseparable from all human relations, language, and thought. This is a central concern and posit of post-modernism thought. The post-modern critique is both a nuisance and uncomfortable for readers and writers, because it does not provide any conceptual wholes as provided by the modernist project. Nursing, by its very nature, helps to determine the culture within which it is practised; it is also very much a product of that culture. As such, nursing is a modernist project primarily concerned with progress. The notions of professionalism and the rise of nursing specialisms are part of the same progress project in which nursing has attempted to create and define a role. Advancement and autonomy are reflections of the ideological and power relations invested in nursing progress. As such, the Advanced Nurse Practitioner (ANP) is seen as the very best the culture of nursing can offer at present. Do you think these are the main points?

Dean: I think these are the important points, but if we consider the sections of this book in sequence, we can give a more detailed overview. I think that in the first section, 'Setting the Modernist Scene', we introduced the idea of 'the self' and 'the power' that psychiatry has in relation to our way of thinking about our current practice; in particular, the notion we have about holism and child-centred care.

Sandy: Did we succeed in our task of introducing the alternative post-modern world view?

Dean: I think our overall task was to highlight that there are alternative ways of thinking about nursing. I think we have succeeded in that. I think we also argued the idea that child and adolescent mental health nursing belongs to a (M)odern world of ideas and is a product of the culture to which it belongs.

Sandy: You mean in the way it assumes Modernist goals to define its role and position in the overall hierarchy? Like the theses about the knowledge base of nursing being fundamentally a modernist concern related to issues of power?

Dean: Exactly, but just as important, I think we acknowledged that these powerful relationships actually contribute to the nature of our practice. The nursing science we all adhere to is a product of our times. If we think about the theses for each of the first three chapters, we can see the way we thought about this late twentieth century position.

Sandy: Well, in The Knowledge Base of Nursing we argued that nursing is Modernist because of its relation to technological, theoretical, and sociological advances; that it cannot be separated from the culture in which it practices.

Dean: The difficulty is defining the inference of progress and Modernity. We argued that the Modernist project of trying to provide a complete and all embracing knowledge base for nursing has failed, because it is an impossible task that nursing has set for itself. This realisation is scary for nursing, and often considered a post-modern flaw. For example, before 1950, nursing believed in the impossible Utopia of an all conclusive knowledge base. It is now perceived by a growing number, that postmodernist critiques has highlighted this impossibility, and also contributed to its realisation.

Sandy: But at least we can begin to acknowledge this and make the best use of the tools we have available to us, such as the therapeutic use of self.

Dean: Yes and no. In *Section I*, we argue that the philosophy of humanism, holism, and systems are seen as fundamental for the scientific and artistic delivery of nursing theory in the care of children. This is, in general, a common assumption, but it draws into the frame once again the concept 'of the self' and each of these philosophies are just ways of 'doing' nursing. They are utilised and well known, because they are the dominant philosophies.

Sandy: The Enlightenment philosophies of humanism and holism, shared by many competing theoretical rivals within health care, merely reflect the way nursing has adopted and is entwined within the Modernist project. Humanism and holism as foundations for practice are ideologically, politically, and culturally determined, even though nursing has invested in them as being scientific and progressive. The idea of 'the use of self' is intrinsic to the way we view child-centred nursing.

Dean: Child-centred caring is a product of our culture. It appeals to our sense of humanity. Unfortunately, it is an idealism rather than a plausible reality. As we discuss throughout the book, there are many different types of forces and powerful constructions, which have a vested interest in expecting the facade of child-centred care, while sustaining the status quo. Child-centred care is what makes child and adolescent nursing unique as a speciality. It provides a platform of specialism and professional role. The fact that this book is concerned with this particular client group emphasises this idea.

Sandy: I think that the arguments we put forward in the second section of the book begin to explore the post-modern issues of representation, reproducibility, and legitimisation, even if this is only at an introductory level.

Dean: I know that the issues of professionalism, ideology, culture, and attachments are just a few out of the many pressing topics that face practitioners, but we had to draw the line somewhere. I think we've managed two things. First, introduced postmodernism to our disciplinary area without necessarily drawing any substantial conclusions. Second, we introduced a new way of viewing our knowledge base.

Sandy: In what way?

Dean: I think the way we have reflected upon the issues presented in Section II has provided a non prescriptive analysis, which may leave the reader feeling cheated.

Sandy: And feeling they haven't really gained anything that can be said to be knowledgeable.

Dean: Exactly, because we have been questioning the very knowledge base from which we practice. This is a critique of the Modernist project; the idea that knowledge can be found and then easily applied to all equally.

Sandy: So why didn't we pick other subjects? I can think of many others, like, assessment, supervision, management issues, risk assessment, and so on...

Dean: Well, you know as well as I do that we could have, and we could have highlighted the cultural and historical context in which all of these and more are considered important. I think that the very fact we are talking about them now illustrates the way the Modernist project is one of many considered 'important topics'. Ten years ago there were other topics. In ten years time there will be more, but the underlying way we view them all will be very much the same. I think that the limited number of topics we have discussed in Section II are the ones that are the broadest for all nurses in child and adolescent mental health.

Sandy: The professionalising of the nursing process being an important one… I'm glad we were able to conclude that it reflects our culture's obsession with order and expected sequences in care provision.

Dean: Well, I think that our exploration of nursing ideology and power relations also emphasised the attention post-modern scholars have paid to these issues. Likewise, the conclusions we drew from the expander/expert chapter emphasises our obsession with defining our role, our power and the boundaries of our practice, as we jostle with other professionals.

Sandy: And the way we do it in terms of attachment theory. Once again, the idea of the 'therapeutic use of self'.

Dean: I wish we could have explored all of these topics in greater detail, but we both know that most of the literature regarding postmodernism is full of difficult and cumbersome terminology. I think that this is a criticism of this section. I think we could have done a better job of explaining some of the terms in more detail, but this would have increased the risk of being even more confusing.

Sandy: But we could say the same about all of the sections. I know that we may have failed in our attempt to convert readers to this broader way of critiquing issues relevant to the Modernist project because of this; but I think we've done a fairly good job of introducing a few of them.

Dean: I think you're right…I think that this section also illustrates how difficult it is entertaining the postmodernist question from the outside. It's very easy to become so tormented with putting the wrongs to right, that you lose all sense of sensibility; and we know by its very nature that our critique throughout *Section II* offers no real solutions; we never intended that.

Sandy: But we have highlighted the way postmodernist thinkers are suspicious of meta-narratives and hierarchies.

Dean: The only consensus being that there can never truly be a consensus regarding the issue of knowledge and power. And the same is true for the issues we introduce in *Section III*.

Sandy: The Postmodernist Project!

Dean: Yes, particularly the idea of authority, containment and the individual, the latter reminding us once again of 'the self'. I think that this section overall begs not the question of how postmodernist thinking can help child and adolescent mental health nursing, but why postmodernism continues to flourish in other academic circles, despite being virtually non existent in nursing?

Sandy: I think we have begun to explore possible reason for this in the postmodernist project section. The idea that we are the product of social constructions and power networks means we maintain a commitment to Modernist values.

Dean: As with the aim of the entire book, we've introduced the idea that it is the understanding of the process and function of the debate, which is just as valuable as its content and outcomes. The way, we have introduced a challenge, albeit a limited one, to the traditional cultural history of nursing ill children, emphasises a new process. We offer no outcomes or solutions, just a new way of re-thinking.

Sandy: By so doing, we have expanded its competency and legitimacy.

Dean: You mean legitimacy being one of the three important concerns in postmodernism critique.

Sandy: I mean, we know that labels, diagnosis, and milieu are products of psychiatric knowledge. They have gained legitimacy through a psychiatric narrative, which emphasises our desire to control and predict that which is considered a natural evil: Madness.

Dean: The idea of the psychiatric narrative is the principle way in which the psychiatric culture legitimises itself. The way we tried to simplify the idea of deconstruction in Section III was not necessarily to be nihilist or undermine psychiatry, but rather, begin a long path towards exploring other world views, perhaps even construct rather than deconstruct.

Sandy: Bearing in mind that one thesis of this book is that both Modernism and postmodernism are self-critical by definition. They legitimise and fool themselves into believing they are self-evaluating and, therefore, more objective.

Dean: Yes, the idea that a global knowledge can be achieved is truly a Modernist project, and postmodernism critique shows that, at a different scale, our culture can become more interested in humans, their symbolic environments, and the construction of the relationships they share. It implies a complete knowledge of the modern that has been surpassed by a new age. There has always been a tension between the past and the present. The history of nursing is made up of many historical and conceptual periods. For example, the Nightingale period, with its concern for clean environments; the supernatural period at the turn of the century; the dominance of the biomedical period; the dawn of the interactional models; and now, 'the anything goes, so long as it is child-centred' period.

IDEOLOGICAL APPOINTMENTS :

(Please note that this Journal can not be held responsible (or perhaps it can) for any ideological or cultural slants it places upon advertisements).

AGENCY ADOLESCENT NURSING AT STRUCTURAL HEIGHTS

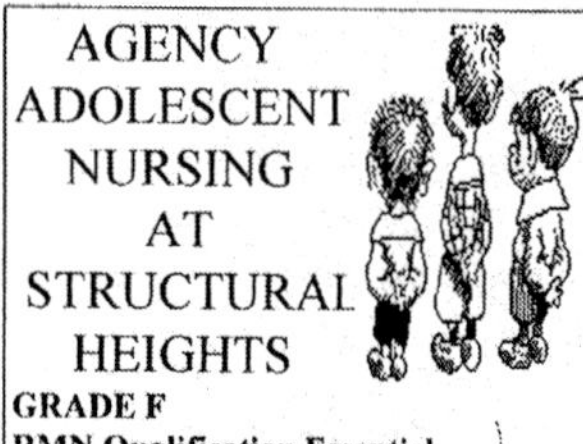

GRADE F
RMN Qualification Essential,
ENB 603 desirable,
2 Years Post Registration Experience.

The Child and Family services are looking for an ideologically determined nurse who has experience with nursing culture to join our team of highly hierarchial and ritualised professionals. The applicant will be able to say 'yes' and appreciate the need for structure in language. No phenomenologists need apply. Contact : J. Derrida, M. Foucault, F. Sassure.

Calling all biologically, medically and behaviourally Modern nurses :

CHILDHOOD LEARNING CENTRE

Grade E.
RMN Essential.

The team is looking for a nurse who is committed to logical ideological reasoning. The cause and effect applicant will be expected to ascertain how ideology and nursing culture can be measured and classified in order to provide predictable patterns. This can be at either a micro or macro level of analysis. The applicant must have a firm commitment to the belief that reality is external to experience and hold a full driving licence. Contact : B. Skinner, E. Goffman, T. Parsons.

WANTED : Old nursing hats, uniforms and aprons. Contact Dean on Ext 4367.

□□□□□□□□□□□

The Ideologically Sound Group Special Offer

Have you ever wondered what it would be like to be a fully trained professional with personal responsibilities ?

Well now you can.

By being a trained nurse you can experience the busy excitment of being involved in the largest systems, care cultures and safe ideologies in the UK.

Just Contact us and have the chance of winning a holiday !

Calling all Phenomenologists :

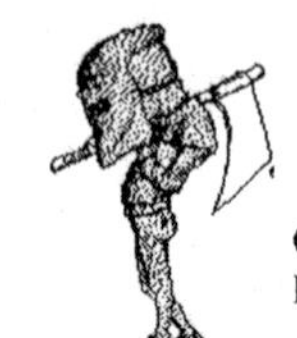

SOLO NHS TRUST
Child & Adolescent Nurses

Grade G Vacancies
RMN / ENB 603 Essential.

The fragmented team is looking for a highly pessimistic existentialist who is capable of working alone within the remit of their monstrous freedom. Their ideology and cultural background must be founded in issues related to humanism, free choice and individual agency. The ideal applicant will assume that nurses are able to deliver totally autonomous care irrespective of the team's ideology and cultural perspective. For a full job description please contact C. Rogers, R.D. Laing or J. Sartre.

74 % of all child and adolescent nurses read this Journal (Honest) and they say it's ideologically sound !

References

Abercrombie N, Hill S, Turner BS (1984) *The Penguin Dictionary of Sociology.* Penguin, Harmondsworth

Addis L (1995) Holism. In: Audi R, ed. *The Cambridge Dictionary of Philosophy.* Cambridge University Press, Cambridge: 336

Agger B (1994) Derrida for sociology? A comment on Fuchs and Ward. *Am Sociolog Rev* **59**: 501–5

Ainsworth MDS (1967) *Infancy in Uganda: Infant Care and the Growth of Love.* Johns Hopkins University Press, Baltimore

Ainsworth MDS (1978) *Patterns of Attachment: A Psychological Study of the Strange Situation.* Lawrence Erlbaum Associates, Hillsdale, NJ

Alexander A, Fawcett J, Runciman P (1995) *Nursing Practice: Hospital and Home The Adult.* Churchill Livingstone, Edinburgh

American Psychiatric Association (1987) *Diagnostic and Statistical Manual of Mental Disorders*, 3rd edn. American Psychiatric Association, Washington DC

American Holistic Nurses Association (1992) Manifesto document. *J Am Holistic Nurses Ass* (September), Sage, California

Andrews S (1989) Specialist or generalist nurse? *Prim Health Care* **6**(2): 8

Appignanesi R, Garratt C (1995) *Postmodernism for Beginners.* ICON Books, Cambridge

Appleton C (1993) The art of nursing: the experience of patients and nurses. *J Adv Nurs* **18**: 892–99

Arena D, Page N (1992) The imposter phenomenon in the CNS role image. *J Nurs Schol* **24**(2): 121–25

Aristotle (1966) Physica. In: Ross WD, ed. Trans. Hardie RP, Gaye RK. *The Works of Aristotle*, Vol 2. Oxford University Press, London: Books i & ii

Bandura A (1986) *Social Foundations of Thought and Action: A Social Cognitive Theory.* Prentice-Hall, Englewood Cliffs, New Jersey

Barker P (1974) *The Residential Work with Children* (rev. edn.) Chaucer Publishing Co, London:

Barker PJ, Reynolds W, Ward T (1995) The proper focus of nursing : a critique of the 'caring' ideology. *Int J Nurs Stud* **32**(4): 386–97

Barthes R (1957) *Mythologies.* Hill and Wang, New York

Bayliss J (1995) Self-care—the ultimate health objective. In: Schober J, Hinchliff S, eds. *Towards Advanced Nursing Practice.* Arnold Press, London: 182–201

Beardshaw V, Robinson M (1990) *New for Old? Prospects for Nursing in the 1990s.* Research Report. King's Fund Institute, London

Beck CK, Rawlins RP, Williams SR (1987) *Mental Health—Psychiatric Nursing: A Holistic Life-Cycle Approach.* The CV Mosby Co, St Louis

Bellack JP, Edlund BJ (1992) *Nursing Assessment and Diagnosis,* 2nd edn. Jones and Bartlett, Boston

Benner P (1984) *From Novice to Expert, Excellence and Power in Clinical Nursing Practice.* Addison Wesley, Menlo Park, California

Benner P, Wrubel J (1989) *The Primacy of Caring: Stress and Coping in Health and Illness.* Addison-Wesley, Menlo Park, California

Berger P (1977) *Pyramids of Power.* Penguin, Harmondsworth

von Bertalanffy L (1968) *General Systems Theory.* Allendale, London

Blackham HJ (1963) Humanism: the subject of the objections. In: Blackham HJ, ed. *Objections to Humanism.* Penguin Books, London: 7–28

Blackham HJ (1963a) The pointlessness of it all. In: Blackham HJ, ed. Objections to Humanism. Penguin Books, London: 103–124

Bowlby J (1980) *Attachment and Loss, Vol 3, Loss, Sadness and Depression.* Hogarth Press, London

Bowlby J (1973) *Attachment and Loss Vol 2, Separation, Anxiety and Anger.* Hogarth Press, London

Bowlby J (1969) *Attachment and Loss, Vol 1, Attachment.* Basic Books, New York

Bowman GS, Thompson DR (1995) Strategies for organising care. In: Schober JE, Hinchcliff SM, eds. *Towards Advancing Nursing Practice.* Arnold, London

Brown PW, Clunn P (1991) Psychiatric hospitals, milieu, and hospital treatment programs. In: Clunn P, ed. *Child Psychiatric Nursing* . Mosby Year Book, St Louis: 435–51

Brykczynska G (1995) Humanism: a weak link in nursing theory? In: Schober JE, Hinchliff SM, eds. *Towards Advanced Nursing Practice.* Arnold, London: 111–32

Buckley W (1967) *Sociology and Modern System Theory.* Prentice-Hall, Englewood Cliffs, NJ

Calkin J (1984) Specialization in nursing practice. In: Baumgort A, Larson J, eds. *Canadian Nursing Faces the Future.* CV Mosby, Toronto: 279–96

Carpenito LT (1995) *Nursing Diagnosis: Application to Clinical Practice,* 6th edn. JB Lippincott, Philadelphia

Carper BA (1978) Fundamental patterns of knowing in nursing. *Adv Nurs Sci* **1**(1): 13–23

Carter H (1994) Confronting patriarchal attitudes in the fight for professional recognition. *J Adv Nurs Pract* **19**: 367–72

Castledine G (1993) Nurse practitioner title: ambiguous and misleading. *Br J Nurs* **2**(14): 734–35

Castledine G (1991a) The advanced nurse practitioner, pt 1. *Nurs Stand* **5**(43): 34–36

Castledine G (1991b) The advanced nurse practitioner, pt 2. *Nurs Stand* **5**(44): 33–35

Chant C (1989) Science and technology: problems of interpretation. In: Chant C, ed. *Science, Technology and Everyday Life 1870–1950.* Open University Press, Milton Keynes: 40–57

Clark E, Gournay K (1995) The individual and health. In: Schober JE, Hinchliff SM, eds. *Towards Advanced Nursing Practice.* Arnold, London: 49–74

Clunn P (1991) *Child Psychiatric Nursing.* Mosby Year Book, St Louis

Coleman R (1998) *Politics of The Madhouse.* Handsell Publishing, Runcorn

Collins J, Mayblin B (1996) *Derrida for Beginners.* Icon Books, Cambridge

Costello AJ (1986) Annotation: assessment and diagnosis of affective disorders in children. *J Child Psychol Psychiatry* **27**(5): 565–74

Crittenden P, Ainsworth MDS (1989) Child maltreatment and attachment theory. In: Cicchetti D, Carlson V, eds. *Handbook of Child Maltreatment: Clinical and Theoretical Perspectives.* Cambridge, New York

Cushing A (1994) Historical and epistemological perspectives on research and nursing. *J Adv Nurs Pract* **20**: 406–11

Department of Health (1994) *'The Heathrow Debate'. Nursing, Midwifery and Health Visiting Education.* Department of Health, HMSO, London

Department of Health and Social Security (1983) *NHS Management Enquiry* (Griffiths Report). HMSO, London

Derrida J (1988) Like the sound of the sea deep within a shell: Paul de Man's War. In: *Memoirs for Paul de Man*, rev edn. Columbia University Press, Columbia

Derrida J (1982) *Margins of Philosophy*, (Bassam A, trans). University of Chicago Press, Chicago

Derrida J (1976) *Of Grammatology*. Johns Hopkins University Press, London/Baltimore

Derrida J (1974) *'Mallarme' in Acts of Literature.* University of Nebraska Press, Nebraska

Derrida J (1973) *Speech and Phenomena, and Other Essays on Husserl's Theory of Signs.* Northwestern University Press, Evanston, IL

Derrida J (1967) *'Differance' in Speech and Phenomena.* Northwest University Press, Illinois

Dickens C (1987) *Hard Times.* Penguin, Middlesex

Draper P (1993) A critique of Fawcett's 'Conceptual models and nursing practice: the reciprocal relationship'. *J Adv Nurs* **18**: 558–64

Drew B (1988) Devaluation of the biological knowledge. *Image* **20**(1): 25–27

Ellis JR, Hartley CL (1992) *Nursing in Today's World—Challenges, Issues and Trends*, 4th edn. JB Lippincott, Philadelphia

Enc B (1995) The paradigm. In: Audi R, ed, *The Cambridge Dictionary of Philosophy.* Cambridge University Press, Cambridge

Erwin E (1997) *Philosophy and Psychotherapy.* Sage, London

Fagin C (1972) *Nursing in Child Psychiatry.* CV Mosby, St Louis

Fann W, Goshen C (1977) *The Language of Mental Health*, 2nd edn. CV Mosby, St Louis

Farlhberg V (1981) *Attachment and Separation* BAAF practice series. Witley Press, Norfolk

Fawcett J (1989) *Analysis and Evaluation of Conceptual Models of Nursing*, 2nd edn. FA Davis, Philadelpia.

Fawcett J (1984) The metaparadigm of nursing: present status and future refinements. *Image* **16**: 84–87

Fawcett J, Downs FS (1992) *The Relationship of Theory and Research*, 2nd edn. FA Davis, Philadelphia

Fay B (1987) *Critical Social Science.* Cornell University Press, Ithaca, NY

Flemming CM (1946) *Adolescence: It's Social Psychology.* Routledge, London

Ford P, Walsh M (1994) *New Rituals for Old.* Butterworth-Heinemann, Oxford

Foucault M (1980) Power/knowledge. *Selected Interviews and Other Writings 1972–1977.* Harvester Press, Brighton

Foucault M (1978) 'About the concept of "Dangerous Individual" in 19th - century legal psychiatry'. *Int J Law Psychiatry* **1**: 1–18

Foucault M (1977) *Discipline and Punish: the Birth of the Prison.* Allen Lane, London

Foucault M (1976) *Mental Illness and Psychology*, (Sheridan A, trans). Harper and Row, New York

Foucault M (1975) *Discipline and Punishment: The Birth of the Prison.* (Sheridan A, trans). Allen Lane (1977), London

Foucault M (1973) *The Order of Things: An Archaeology of the Human Sciences*, (Trans. Non-listed). Random House Vintage Books, New York

Foucault M (1971) *Madness and Civilization.* Tavistock, London

Foucault, M (1967) *Madness and Civilization: A History of Insanity in the Age of Reason.* Tavistock, London

Freud S (1997) *The Interpretation of Dreams.* (Brill AA, trans). Wordsworth Classics, Hertfordshire

Fuchs S, Ward S (1994) What is deconstruction, and where and when does it take place? Making facts in science, building cases in law. *Am Sociolog Rev* **59**: 481–500

Gavin JN (1997) Nursing ideology and the 'generic carer'. *J Adv Nurs* **26**: 692–97

Giddens A (1993) *Sociology*, 2nd edn. Polity Press, Cambridge

Goffman E (1961) *Asylums.* Anchor Books, Doubleday & Co, New York, (Pelican Books, Middlesex (1968))

Gortner SR (1990) Nursing values and science: toward a science philosophy. *Image: J Nurs Schol* **22**(2): 101–5

Gray G, Pratt R eds (1991) Prologue. In: *Towards a Discipline of Nursing.* Churchill Livingstone, London: 1–9

Greenburg C (1980) The Notion of 'Post-Modern'. *4th Sir William Dotell Memorial Lecture.* University of Sydney. Bloxham and Chambers

Grossmann KE, Grossmann K (1990) The Wider concept of attachment in cross-cultural research. *Hum Devel* **33**: 31–47

Habermas J (1971) *Knowledge and Human Interests.* (Shapiro JJ, trans) Beacon Press, Boston, MA

Hall C (1990) *Health and the Global Environment.* Polity Press, Cambridge

Hamilton PM (1992) *Realities of Contemporary Nursing.* Addison-Wesley Nursing, New York

Haraway D (1988) Situated knowledges: The science question in feminism and the privilege of partial perspective. *Fem Stud* **14**(3): 576–99

Harwood RL, Miller JG, Irizarry NL (1995) *Culture and Attachment: Perceptions of the Child in Context.* Guilford Press, London

HAS Report (1995) *Child and Adolescent Mental Health Services.* The NHS Health Advisory Service. HMSO, London

Hector W (1982) *Modern Nursing: Theory and Practice.* Heinemann, London

Heidegger M (1962) *Being and Time*, (Macquarrie J, Robinson E, trans). Harper & Row, New York

Heidegger M (1958) *What is Philosophy*? (Kluback W, Wilde J, trans) Twayne, New York

Heideman J, Crabbe V (1991) Historical overview and current status of child psychiatric nursing. In: Clunn P, ed. *Child Psychiatric Nursing.* Mosby Year Book, St Louis: 3–13

Heider F (1958) *The Psychology of Interpersonal Relations.* John Wiley, New York

Henderson A (1994) Power and knowledge in nursing practice: the contribution of Foucault. *J Adv Nurs* **20**: 935–39

Hepworth J (1994) Qualitative analysis and eating disorders: discourse analytic research on anorexia nervosa. *Int J Eat Disord* **15**: 179–85

Herbert M (1988) *Working With Children and Their Families.* Routledge, London

Hewison A (1995) Nurses' power in interactions with patients. *J Adv Pract* **21**: 75–82

Hilton PA (1997) Theoretical perspectives of nursing: a review of the literature. *J Adv Nurs* **26**: 1211–20

Hinchliff SM, Norman SE, Schober JE (1993) *Nursing Practice and Health Care.* Edward Arnold, London

Hoare P (1993) *Essential Child Psychiatry.* Churchill Livingstone, London

Hogston R (1997) Nursing diagnosis and classification systems: a position paper. *J Adv Nurs* **26**: 496–500

Hollinger R (1994) *Postmodernism in the Social Sciences: A Thermetic Approach.* Sage, Thousand Oaks, California

Holmes J (1993) *John Bowlby and Attachment Theory.* Routledge, London

Holyoake D (1999) Favourite patients: exploring labelling in inpatient culture. *Nurs Stand* **13**(16): 44–47

Holyoake D (1998a) Advanced nursing practice in a culture of mental health nursing. In: Thorbrook P, Rolfe G, eds. *Perspectives of Advanced Nursing Practice*, University of Portsmouth (April, 1988)

Holyoake D (1998b) Reflections on the process of play interaction. *Paediatr Nurs* **10**(2): 14–17

Holyoake D (1998c) Disentangling caring from love in a nurse-patient relationship. *Nurs Times* **94**(49): 56–59

Holyoake D (1998d) Observing nurse-patient interaction. *Nurs Stand* **12**(29): 35–37

Holyoake D (1997a) A look into the culture club: Exploring the perceptions of mentally ill young people about in-patient culture. *Psychiatr Care* **4**(3): 162–67

Holyoake D (1997b) Philosophy of the culture club: exploring the philosophical basis of nursing mentally ill young people. *Paediatr Nurs* **9**(8): 18–21

Holyoake D (1995) Advancing in confusion. *Nurs Stand* **9**(51): 56

Hopton J (1997) Towards a critical theory of mental health nursing. *J Adv Nurs* **25**: 492–500

Hopton J (1993) The contradictions of mental health nursing. *Nurs Stand* **8**(11): 37–39

Husserl E (1982) *General Introduction to a Pure Phenomenology.* (Kersten F, trans). Martinus Nijhoff, The Hague

Jacono B, Jacono J (1994) Power tactics and their potential impact on nursing. *J Adv Nurs* **19**: 954–59

Johnson C (1997) *Derrida.* Orion Publishing Group, London

Johnson FC, Smith LD (1994) Personal and professional roles, skills and behaviours: present and future. In: Thompson T, Mathias P, eds.

Lyttle's Mental Health and Disorder, 2nd edn. Bailliere Tindall, London: 12–40

Jones K (1991) The culture of the mental hospital. In: Berrios GE, Freeman H, eds. *150 Years of British Psychiatry 1841–1991*. Gaskell, London

Jones L (1994) *The Social Context of Health and Health Work*. Macmillan, London

Jones M (1953) *The Therapeutic Community: A Treatment Method in Psychiatry*. Basic Books, New York

Joseph D (1985) Humanism: as a philosophy for nursing. *Nurs For* **xxii**(4): 135–38

Kant I (1785; 1956) *Groundwork of the Metaphysic of Morals*, (Paton HJ, trans). Harper, London

Kataoka-Yahiro M, Saylor C (1994 A critical thinking model for nursing judgement. *J Nurs Educ* **33**: 351–56

Kikuchi J, Simmons H (1992) *Philosophic Inquiry in Nursing*. Sage, Newbury Park

Kitson A (1993) Formalising concepts related to nursing and caring. In: Kitson A, ed. *Nursing Art and Science*. Chapman & Hall, London: 25–47

Kolcaba R (1997) The primary holisms in nursing. *J Adv Nurs* **25**(2): 290–96

Kolenda K (1995) Humanism. In: *The Cambridge Dictionary of Philosophy*. Cambridge University Press, Cambridge: 340–41

Kramer MK (1990) Holistic nursing: implications for knowledge development and utilisation. In: Chaska NL, ed. *The Nursing Profession. Turning Points*. CV Mosby, St Louis: 245–54

Kubsch SM (1996) Conflict, enactment, empowerment: conditions of independent therapeutic nursing intervention. *J Adv Nurs* **23**: 192–200

Kuhn T (1962/1977) *The Structure of Scientific Revolutions*, 2nd edn. The University of Chicago Press, Chicago, IL

Kuhn TS (1970) *The Structure of Scientific Revolutions*. University of Chicago Press, Chicago

Kvale S (1990) Introduction. In: Kvale S, ed. *Psychology and Postmodernism*. Sage Publications, London: 1–16

Lather P (1990) Postmodernism and the human sciences. In: Kvale S, ed. *Psychology and Postmodernism*. Sage Publications, London: 88–109

Layton ET, Jr (1977) Conditions of technological development. In: Spiegel-Rosing I, Price DJ de S, eds. *Science, Technology and Society: A Cross-Disciplinary Perspective.* Sage, London: 197–222

Lechte J (1994) *Fifty Key Contemporary Thinkers: From Structuralism to Postmodernity.* Routledge, London

Levin L (1981) Self-care: towards fundamental changes in national strategies. *Int J Health Educ* **24**: 4

Lister P (1997) The art of nursing in a 'postmodern' context. *J Adv Nurs* **25**: 38–44

Lovlie L (1990) Postmodernism and subjectivity. In: Kvale S, ed. *Psychology and Postmodernism.* Sage Publications, London: 119–34

Lutzen K, Tishelman C (1996) Nursing diagnosis: a critical analysis of underlying assumptions. *Int J Nurs Stud* **33**(2): 190–200

Lyotard JF (1984) *The Postmodern Condition: A Report on Knowledge.* (Bennington G, Massumi B, trans.) University of Minnesota Press, Minneapolis

MacDonald KM (1995) *The Sociology of the Professions.* Sage, London

McGee P (1993) Defining nursing practice. *Br J Nurs* **2**(20): 1022–26

McInerny R (1995) 'Postmodern'. In: *The Cambridge Dictionary of Philosophy.* Cambridge University Press, Cambridge: 634

Marcuse HG (1982) Ethnographics as text. *Ann Rev Anthropol* **11**: 25–69

Marris P (1991) The social construction of uncertainty. In: Parkes CM, Stevenson-Hinde J, eds. *Attachment across the Life Cycle.* Routledge, London

Maslow AH (1970) *Motivation and Personality*, 2nd edn. Harper & Row, New York

Masson J (1990) *Against Therapy.* Harper Collins Publishers, London

Merleau-Ponty M (1948) *Sense and Non-Sense*, (Dryfus HL, Dryfus PA, trans). Northwestern University Press, Evanston (1964)

Michael M (1990) Postmodern subjects: towards a transgressive social psychology. In: Kvale S, ed. *Psychology and Postmodernism.* Sage Publications. London: 74–87

Miller J (1965) Living systems: Basic concepts. *Behav Sci* **10**: 93–237

Moore JR (1989) Everyday life and the dynamics of technological change. In: Chant C, ed. *Science, Technology and Everyday Life 1870–1950.* Open University Press, Milton Keynes: 9–39

Morse J (1989) Qualitative nursing research: a free for all? In: Morse J, ed. *Qualitative Nursing Research: A Contemporary Dialogue.* Aspen Publishers, Rockville, Maryland: 3–10

Moser PK (1995) Foundationalism. In: *The Cambridge Dictionary of Philosophy.* Cambridge University Press, Cambridge: 276–78

Murphy JF (1970) Role expansion or role extension. *Nurs Forum* **9**(4): 380–90; 494–501

Nolan P (1993) *A History of Mental Health Nursing.* Chapman and Hall, London

Norris C (1987) *Derrida.* Fontana, London

North American Nursing Diagnosis Association (NANDA) (1990) NANDA Definition. *Nurs Diag* **1**(2): 50

Ogbu JU (1981) Origins of human competence: A cultural-ecological perspective. *Child Devel* **52**: 413–29

Onega LL (1991) A theoretical framework for psychiatric nursing practice. *J Adv Nurs* **16**: 68–73

Orem D (1991) *Nursing Concepts of Practice*, 4th edn. Mosby Year Book, St Louis

Osbourne R, Edney R (1992) *Philosophy for Beginners.* Writers and Readers Books, New York

Packard SA, Polifroni EC (1991) The dilemma of nursing science: current quandaries and lack of direction. *Nurs Sci Q* **4**(1): 7–13

Paice R (1996) Nursing in a child psychiatric unit. In: Chesson R, Chisholm D, eds. *Child Psychiatric Units At the Crossroads.* Jessica Kingsley, London

Palmer DD (1997) *Structuralism and Poststructuralism for Beginners.* Writers and Readers Books, New York

Parker I, Georgaca E, Harper D, McLaughlin T, Stowell-Smith M (1995) *Deconstructing Psychopathology.* Sage, London

Parse RR (1981) *Man-Living-Health: A Theory of Nursing.* John Wiley & Sons, New York

Parsons T (1951) *The Social System.* Routledge, London & New York

Pasquali EA, Arnold HM, DeBasio N (1989) *Mental Health Nursing: A Holistic Approach*, 3rd edn. CV Mosby Company, St Louis

Paterson JG, Zderad LT (1988) *Humanistic Nursing.* National League for Nursing, New York

Patterson C, Haddad B (1992) The advanced nurse practitioner: common attributes. *Can J Nurs Admin* **Nov/Dec**: 18–20

Peplau H (1989) Future directions in psychiatric nursing from a perspective of history. *J Psychosoc Nurs Mental Health Serv* **27**(21): ??pp nos??

Peplau HE (1952/1988) *Interpersonal Relations in Nursing*, 2nd edn. Macmillan Press, London

Perlmutter H, Trist E (1986) *Paradigms for Societal Transition.* Tavistock Institute of Human Relations, London

Plato (1968) Timaeus. In: *Dialogues of Plato*, Vol 3 (Jowett B, trans). Oxford University Press, London

Playle JF (1995) Humanism and positivism in nursing: Contradictions and conflicts. *J Adv Nurs* **22**: 979–89

Plotz P (1988) The disappearance of childhood: parent-child role reversals in after the first death and solitary blue. *Children's Lit Educ* **19**: 67

Popper KR (1959) *The Logic of Scientific Discovery.* Hutchinson, London

Pursey M (1994) Suicide, explanation and moral reasoning. Unpublished M.Litt thesis, University of Birmingham

Quay HC, Peterson DR (1984) Interim manual for the revised behavior problem checklist. Unpublished manuscript

Rafferty D (1991) Of primary importance. *Sen Nurse* **11**(6): 4–8

Ray M (1991) Caring inquiry: the aesthetic process in the way of compassion. In: Gaut DA, Leininger MM, eds. *Caring: The Compassionate Healer.* National League for Nursing, New York: 123–33

Ray M (1990) Phenomenological method of nursing research. In: Chaska N, ed. *The Nursing Profession: Turning Point.* McGraw Hill, New York: 173–78

Reeves M (1946) *Growing Up in a Modern Society.* London University Press, London

Rey JM, Plapp JM, Stewart GW (1989) Reliability of psychiatric diagnosis in referred adolescents. *J Child Psychol Psychiatry* **30**(6): 879–88

Richer P (1990) An introduction to deconstructing psychology. In: Kvale S, ed. *Psychology and Postmodernism.* Sage Publications, London:110–18

Rizzo AE, Ossorio A, Saxon L (1986) The organization of an adolescent unit in a state hospital: Problems and attempted solutions. In: Sugar M, ed. *The Adolescent in Group and Family Therapy*, 2nd edn. University of Chicago Press, Chicago: 68–86

Robertson J (1952) Film: *A Two-Year-Old Goes to Hospital.* Tavistock, London

Rogers C (1951) *Client-centered Therapy: Its Current Practice, Implications and Theory.* Houghton Mifflin, Boston

Rogers C, Stevens B (1971) *Person to Person: The Problem of Being Human.* Pocket Books, New York

Rogers ME (1970) *An Introduction to the Theoretical Basis of Nursing.* FA Davis, Philadelphia

Roper N (1988) *Principles of Nursing in Process Context.* Churchill Livingstone, Edinburgh

Rowe D (1990) Forward to against therapy. In: Mason J, ed. *Against Therapy.* Harper-Collins Publishers, London: 7–23

Royal College of Nursing (1988) *Specialities in Nursing.* RCN, London

Rushing B (1993) Ideology in the re-emergence of North American midwifery. *Work Occupat* **20**(1): 46–67

Rutter M (1989) Annotation: child psychiatric disorders in ICD-10. *J Child Psychol Psychiatry* **30**(4): 499–513

Rutty JE (1998) The nature of philosophy of science, theory and knowledge relating to nursing and professionalism. *J Adv Nurs* **28**(2): 243–50

Sartre JP (1992) *Being and Nothingness,* (Barnes H, trans). Washington Square Press, New York

Sartre JP (1990) *Being and Nothingness: Essays on Phenomenological Ontology.* Routledge, London

Sarup M (1988) *Post-Structuralism and Post-Modernism.* Harvester Wheatsheaf, London

Saussure F (1994) *Course in General Linguistics,* (Harris R, trans). Lasalle, Illinois

Schober J (1995) Nursing: current issues and the patient's perspective. In: Schober JE, Hinchliff SM, eds. *Towards Advanced Nursing Practice.* Arnold, London: 75–110

Skinner BF (1953) *Science and Human Behaviour.* Macmillan, New York

Skinner BF (1938) *The Behaviour of Organisms.* Appleton-Century-Crofts, New York

Smith R (1997) *The Fontana History of the Human Sciences.* Fontana Press, London

Smuts JC (1926) *Holism and Evolution.* Macmillan, New York

Sparacino P (1992) Advanced practice: the clinical nurse specialist. *Nurse Practit* **5**(4): 2–4

Steinberg D (1987) *Basic Adolescent Psychiatry*. Blackwell Scientific Publications, London

Stensrud RH (1984) Holistic health. In: Corsini RJ, ed. *Encyclopeadia of Psychology*, 2nd edn, Vol 2. John Wiley & Sons, New York: 146–49

Strauss CL (1978) *Introduction to a Science of Mythology Vol 1: The Raw and the Cooked*, (Weightman J, Weightman D, trans). Jonathon Cape, London

Strauss CL (1964) *Tristes Tropiques*, (Russell J, trans). Atheneum, New York

Suominen T, Kovasin M, Ketola O (1997) Nursing culture—some viewpoints. *J Adv Nurs* **25**: 186–90

Symington R (1997) Inadequate and patchy: mental health services for children and young people. *Mental Health: The Newsletter for Nurses Working in Mental Health* (Winter). RCN, London: 9

Szasz T (1961) *The Myth of Mental Illness.* Harper and Row, New York.

Taylor F (1911) *The Principles of Scientific Measurement.* Harper & Row, London

Taylor JS (1997) Nursing ideology: identification and legitimation. *J Adv Nurs* **25**: 442–46

The Children Act (1989) *An Introductory Guide for the NHS.* DoH, London

Therborn G (1980) *The Ideology of Power and the Power of Ideology.* New Left Books, London

Thompson JB (1990) *Ideology and Modern Culture.* Polity Press, Cambridge

Thompson K (1986) *Beliefs and Ideology.* Tavistock, London

Thompson T, Mathias P (1994) The core concepts of care in mental health and disorder. In: Thompson T, Mathias P, eds. *Lyttle's Mental Health and Disorder*, 2nd edn. Bailliere Tindall, London: 7–11

Thornbory G, Murugiah S (1995) Environment and health. In: Schober J, Hinchliff S, eds. *Towards Advanced Nursing Practice.* Arnold Press, London: 29–48

Timpson J (1996) Nursing theory: everything the artist spits is art? *J Adv Nurs* **23**: 1030–36

Trnobranski P (1993) Biological sciences and the nursing curriculum: a challenge for educationalists. *J Adv Nurs* **18**: 493–99

United Kingdom Central Council for Nursing, Midwifery and Health Visiting (1997) *UKCC's Position on Advanced Practice.* Press Statement 8/1997 UKCC, London.

United Kingdom Central Council for Nursing, Midwifery and Health Visiting (1994) *The Future of Professional Practice. The Council's Standards for Education and Practice Following Registration.* UKCC, London

United Kingdom Central Council for Nursing, Midwifery and Health Visiting (1993) *The Council's Proposed Standards for Post-Registration Education.* UKCC, London

United Kingdom Central Council for Nursing, Midwifery and Health Visiting (1992) *The Scope of Professional Practice.* UKCC, London

United Kingdom Central Council for Nursing, Midwifery and Health Visiting (1990) *The Report of the Post-Registration Education and Practice Project.* UKCC, London

Vitello-Cicciu J (1984) Excellence in critical care: educating the clinical specialist. *Crit Care Q* **7**(1): 26–32

Watson J (1988) *Nursing. Human Science and Human Care: A Theory of Nursing.* National League for Nursing, New York

Watson J, Rayner R (1920) Conditioned emotional reactions. *J Exper Psychol* **3**(1): 415

Watson JB (1983) *Psychology from the Standpoint of a Behaviourist*, 2nd edn. NH Frances Pinter, London and Dover

Wheeler SC (1995) Deconstruction. In: *The Cambridge Dictionary of Philosophy.* Cambridge University Press, Cambridge: 181–82

White A (1993) *Management for Clinicians.* Edward Arnold, London

Williams FS (1986) Family therapy: its role in adolescent psychiatry. In: Sugar M, ed. *The Adolescent in Group and Family Therapy*, 2nd edn. The University of Chicago Press, Chicago: 178–93

Williams R (1976) *Keywords.* Fontana, London

Winnicot D (1990) *Maturational Processes and the Facilitating Environment.* Hogarth Press, London

Witz A (1991) *Professions and Patriarchy.* Routledge, London

Wood D ed (1992) *Derrida: A Critical Reader.* Blackwell, Oxford

Wood G (1983) *The Myth of Neurosis.* Macmillan, London

Wynne N, Brand S, Smith R (1997) Incomplete holism in pre-registration nurse education: the position of the biological sciences. *J Adv Nurs* **26**(3): 470–74

Index